SHANNON MCRAE, PHD

with

SCOTT E. MINERS

The Healing Effects of ENERGY MEDICINE

MEMOIRS OF A MEDICAL INTUITIVE

Foreword by

BERNIE SIEGEL, MD

New Age Books

New Delhi (India)

THE HEALING EFFECTS OF ENERGY MEDICINE

MEMOIRS OF A MEDICAL INTUITIVE

ISBN: 978-81-7822-494-7

First Indian Edition: Delhi, 2017
First USA Edition: 2015

(Published by arrangement with the Theosophical Publishing House, 306 West Geneva Road, Wheaton, IL, 60187, U.S.A.)

Published by
NEW AGE BOOKS
A-44 Naraina Industrial Area, Phase-I
New Delhi (India) 110028
E-mail: nab@newagebooksindia.com
Website: www.newagebooksindia.com

Library of Congress Cataloging-in-Publication Data
McRae, Shannon
ISBN 978-81-7822-494-7
Includes Foreword, Prologue, Introduction, Notes, Index
Healing/Health

For Sale in Indian Sub-continent Only.

Printed and published by
RP Jain for NAB Printing Unit
A-44, Naraina Industrial Area
Phase-I, New Delhi-110028. India
Printed at: Ar Emm International, Delhi.

I dedicate this book to all my clients who have worked through the years to improve their lives; to the many researchers and authors who have preceded me and discovered ways to explain energy medicine, energy fields, and how thought and intent play such an important role in health; to Scott Miners for his undying faith and belief in me; and to my family for shaping me through my early childhood experiences and unknowingly pushing me deeply to understand myself and my surroundings. I offer this book to help you, the reader, to a greater self-understanding, and hope you will find something in it that will improve your life.

—Shannon McRae

I dedicate my work here to all my relations everywhere, especially to my father, who taught me to leave the campsite in better shape than when I arrived; and to my mother, who showed me that you can't know how much love there is in others until you look.

—Scott E. Miners

Try and be a sheet of paper with nothing on it.
Be a spot of ground where nothing is growing,
where something might be planted,
a seed, possibly, from the Absolute.

—Jalal al-Din Rumi

Contents

	Foreword by Bernie Siegel, MD	**xi**
	Prologue by Scott E. Miners	**xvii**
	Preface	**xxiii**
	Introduction: The Girl Who Could See What Others Could Not	**1**
1	Cellular Healing, Quantum Things, and Our Organizational DNA	**15**
2	Healing an Arterial Tear, Genetic Potential, and Removing Cancer Cells	**29**
3	Healing Cells and Repairing an Eardrum	**37**
4	Presence, Prayer, and Healing a Headache	**43**
5	Unconditional Desire and Healing a Wound	**49**
6	Self-Worth, Thoughts, Beliefs, and Stress	**53**
7	A Case Demonstrating the Reversal of Cellular Stress: The Importance of Positive Thought and Emotion	**61**
8	Old Beliefs, Emotions, and Intuitional Perception for Healing	**69**

9 The Importance of Letting Go of Unwanted Conditions 73

10 The Healing Power of Forgiveness 75

11 Anxiety, Depression, and the Power of Talk Therapy with Energy Medicine 81

12 Beyond Ego, Forgiveness, and the Power of Ease 89

13 Our Bodies and the Profound Health Effects of Appreciation 97

14 Healing Cancer with Energy Medicine 101

15 Being Unconditionally Present as Part of the Healing Process 113

16 Healing by Letting Go of Emotional Pain 119

17 The Energies of Emotions and Their Effects on the Body 125

18 Coherence and Unexpected Healing 131

19 Intent, Focus, and Healing over a Long Distance: Positive Thought, Presence, and a Case of Healing the Lungs 141

20 Hepatitis C, Energy Medicine, and Turning a Challenge into a Success Story 149

21 Healing Emotional Conditions 155

22 The Importance of Alignment with Healing 159

23 Resolving Conflicting Beliefs 163

24	Obsessive-Compulsive Behavior and How Feeling Good Enough Opens the Doors to Healing	**169**
25	Resilience and Forgiveness: Keys to Health	**173**
26	A Case of Sinus Pain and Infections	**177**
27	Boundaries, Allowing, and Complete Health	**181**
	Epilogue: Life after Life and Unseen Helpers	**189**
	Index	**215**

Foreword

The gift of unbearable need is such that those who have suffered a loss, especially in childhood, are especially gifted in unusual ways.

—LAURA DAY, *How to Rule the World from Your Couch*

Having experienced the energy medicine that Shannon McRae describes, I accept what I know to be true even if I can't explain it. Like Albert Einstein, I believe that everything is a miracle and that all living things have incredible innate potential. Science often functions with a closed mind, is based upon limited beliefs, and ignores the kinds of experiences Shannon describes in which she uses her intuition and channels healing energies to help restore others to health. Science, because it cannot explain such healings, in general refuses to do research related to them.

In a way similar to Shannon's seminal near-death experience (NDE) as a child, I had an early-life NDE that showed me that there is more to living than we can perceive with our five senses. When I was four years old I was home in bed with one of my frequent ear infections. I unscrewed the dial on a toy telephone and put all the pieces in my mouth, just as I had seen carpenters do with nails that they pulled out to reuse. The problem was that I aspirated the pieces and went into laryngospasm. My intercostal muscles and diaphragm contracted forcefully, trying to get some air into my lungs, but nothing worked, and I was unable to call for help. I had no sense of the time but suddenly realized I was not struggling anymore. I was now at the head of the bed watching myself dying.

During my NDE I found it fascinating and a blessing to be free of my four-year-old body. I never stopped to wonder about how I could still see and think while out of my body, but in remembering the event, I know that I could. At the time, my mother was in the kitchen. I felt sorry for her and feared her finding me dead. But thinking it over, I found my new state preferable, so intellectually I chose death over life in my body.

Then I watched myself as the four-year-old boy on the bed vomited. All the toy pieces came flying out, and he began to breathe again. I was very angry as I returned to my body, seemingly against my will. I can still remember yelling, "Who did that?" In recalling the event later, I began to think that there was a God who had a plan and that I hadn't been supposed to die yet. The way I would explain the experience today is that an angel had done a Heimlich maneuver on me. Shannon describes silvery beings who comforted her when she was sick as a child, and I think these unseen helpers are there for all of us.

Later in life, as a practicing physician, I was at an American Holistic Medical Association conference where the healer Olga Worrall was a guest speaker. I had just injured my leg while training for a marathon. It was very painful and not responding to rest or therapy. My wife told me to ask Olga, after her presentation, to heal me. I was embarrassed to ask and, very frankly, a non-believer. Nevertheless, my wife pushed me forward, and Olga sat me down in a chair and placed her two hands on my leg. The heat from her hands was incredible. I remember putting my hands on my other leg to compare the heat sensation. There was no sense of warmth coming from my hands through the dungarees. When Olga was finished, I stood up and was completely healed. The pain was gone, and I could walk normally. That the same healing energy comes through Shannon therefore does not surprise me. Nor am I surprised that her many clients often say they can feel warmth or tingling sensations, or even that she can conduct this healing energy long distance over the phone, as well. Her powerful stories in this book are proof that unseen energies of healing are perpetually accessible.

Shannon's descriptions of being able to see intuitively remind me of a number of such events I have experienced myself, with my patients as well as in my private life. One time, for example, Olga and I spoke at the funeral of a mutual friend. After the ceremony, we were standing in a deserted hallway when she asked, "Are you Jewish?"

"Why are you asking?" I said.

"Because there are two rabbis standing next to you." She went on to tell me their names and describe their garments, which included their prayer shawls and caps. Her description of them was exactly what I saw in my meditation and imagery sessions, where I had perceived these figures as inner guides.

On another occasion, as I gave a lecture, it felt like someone else was giving it. I simply verbalized the thoughts that came to me. Afterward, a woman came up to me and said, "Standing in front of you for the entire lecture was a certain man in spirit, and I drew his picture for you." She had drawn exactly as I had pictured before, in my mind, the face and features of one of my inner guides. I have the picture hanging in our home.

Such experiences confirm for me the certainty that Shannon's ability to perceive unseen helpers and communicate with them can be very healing for those who seek her help. We all are more connected to the unseen world than we know.

From my experience with animal communication and other experiences like them, I am also certain that consciousness is nonlocal and not limited to the body. Shannon's healing stories in this book show that something unlimited is helping us all heal and be in health. I have seen healings like those she describes that first were depicted through the drawings and dreams of my patients. These drawings have allowed them to know their diagnoses beyond the intellect and beyond conventional medicine; often the drawings and dreams even describe what the future holds for my patients. Depth psychologist C. G. Jung said, "The future is unconsciously prepared long in advance and therefore can be guessed by clairvoyants." I believe such awareness—as you will see emerged so clearly for Shannon—is something we are all imbued with at birth.

The intelligent, conscious, loving energy of creation is available to us all if we can quiet our minds and sense the connection between the universal and our own individual consciousness. The healings Shannon describes bring our attention to this universal energy of well-being that is flowing to and through us at all times. I remember once when my children refused to let me have our veterinarian euthanize our dog Oscar, who had extensive metastatic melanoma. The vet felt the dog would never recover. I brought Oscar home, laid him on the floor, and every day shared my meals, vitamins, and love with him; I did the latter by the laying on of hands and by massaging him whenever I had a free moment. In two weeks he was on his feet and running around; he lived for three more years with no sign of cancer—a fact that left our veterinarian amazed.

As Shannon notes, for our healing and our everyday lives, it is important that we attune to the coherence of our existence. We need to heighten our awareness of the continuous power for healing that flows to both our physical and spiritual aspects and of the intelligence coming to us through each. So much of what we call well-being flows to us in unseen ways. For example, the day of my father's death, a voice I heard in my mind asked me, "How did your parents meet?" I said I didn't know, and the voice said, "Then ask your mother when you get to the hospital." I did so, and the stories my mother told allowed my dad to die laughing. In another example, when I finished writing a book called *Buddy's Candle,* I heard a voice advise me to go to the animal shelter. I did, and when I walked in I saw a dog sitting by the door. I asked for his name, and the shelter worker said, "His name is Buddy. He has been here less than fifteen minutes." I adopted Buddy that day. Buddy, just as with all good animals, provides his constant, natural healing flow of energy in our household.

Shannon mentions the importance of the patient needing to be part of the healing, and I agree. We need to open our minds and explore the potential of energy medicine to transform our lives and bring about "self-induced healing," as Alexander Solzhenitsyn puts it in his book *Cancer Ward.* We must have hope. There is no physician, no healer, who can help patients if those patients are not determined to participate in the healing themselves.

Healing is not a spontaneous remission or a miracle; it involves the intention of the person being healed. A patient has to cooperate to create harmony and rhythm and transform his or her formerly ill self into one with wellness; if we focus and listen, there are messages being communicated to each of us from our minds and bodies. The messages I heard in my mind are only two examples of the many ways we can discern transformative messages. I can help a patient as a physician, and a healer such as Shannon can, too, but as Shannon states, patients have to love their lives and bodies in order to facilitate the self-healing, as well. Because of my experiences, I have no doubt about Shannon's intuitive sense of knowing what is causing a disease for someone and her remarkable abilities to help so many people heal from their ills.

—Bernie Siegel, MD

Prologue

Intuition is like when you know something,but like, where did it come from?

—A fifteen-year-old girl's definition of intuition, from Lynn Robinson's *Divine Intuition*

Shannon McRae earned a PhD in psychology early in her life and has long practiced and helped thousands of clients. However, her experiences and work with intuition and healing, too, are notable. Her natural intuitive skills have always been a part of her practice, but here the focus is on a close view as to just how accurate she is and how she uses her intuitive insight to help her clients.

The world of medicine is no stranger to the insights of intuition and the healing power of touch and intention. Shannon early on dedicated her life to assisting and serving others; that is her main focus, from the way she interacts with others daily—shopping, driving, paying the bills, dining out, traveling, visiting, attending concerts—to the way she focuses on helping her clients day in and day out. Some might call it naïve to live the way she lives, always ready to assist another, but the results of her life speak rather to a loving, healing, and masterful one. She lives a healing life, and her essence is one of being almost always tuned in, tapped in, and turned on to the subtle healing energies that are flowing to all of us.

I had known Shannon as a friend for many years before I knew about her intuitive insights, and even then I learned about them only through her husband, David, who had also become a wonderful friend. Shannon did not talk about her abilities, but David told me about what she did for others and the remarkable insights she has that some would call *psychic*, but that here we are calling *intuitive*.

After David's disclosures, I wanted to know more. The first thing I did after learning about her insights and healing work was to ask her to help me heal from an irritating skin cancer. She did so; the cancer healed and was gone almost overnight. I then wanted to know much more about what happened and how she knew what she knew. She told me things that truly opened my eyes. That story was published in the *Well Being Journal*, and, in more concise form, is included in this book. Shannon has an extraordinary ability and life that hardly anyone ever sees; however, her many clients all over the world whom she has helped heal from their illnesses, both physical and emotional, can testify on her behalf.

As I began to learn more about Shannon and her work, I wanted to present her healing stories in the *Well Being Journal*. As editor of the *Journal*, I met regularly with her to edit notes and drafts of her writing containing her experiences. Through the years, I had to ask her innumerable questions, because all that her drafts contained were notes and comments about her clients, such as, "Henry M. called and I helped him heal his cancer over several sessions." When I asked how she had accomplished the healing, she would smile and say, "Oh, I just do what I do." But then I would reply, most calmly, "Can you say just a little more?" I continually had to ask, "How did you do that? See that? Know that?" As the months and years rolled by, I came to realize the easy insight she has into disease and health processes—that is, easy for her, but remarkable to those of us who have not practiced the openness to subtle ways of knowing that she has.

Shannon does not seem to give much thought to the fact that her insights and healing abilities are out of the ordinary, because they have come naturally to her all her life. Since my work calls me to write extensively and edit others' writing as well, I found it easy to compose stories while Shannon answered my questions and described her client cases. Roberta Louis and I then edited the material, and Shannon proofread, making changes here and there. Then we went to press with her articles, tailored to a general reading audience, in the *Well Being Journal.* Most of the chapters that follow consist of those articles, revised for this book.

I began to learn about therapeutic touch, energy medicine, intuitive medicine, and clairvoyance in medicine in the late 1970s through working with the medical clairvoyant Dora van Gelder Kunz, the executive editor of *The American Theosophist* and the cofounder, along with Dolores Krieger, of therapeutic touch. Dora worked all her long life with many physicians, health professionals, and scientists worldwide—Shafica Karagulla, Bernie Siegel, Larry Dossey, Fritjof Capra, and Mael Melvin, to name just a few—who were fascinated by the field of energy medicine. While working as Dora's managing editor at the time, I benefited by being able and willing to learn as much as I could. These professionals were then discussing the evidence that the solid physical world, and therefore medicine itself, was underpinned by the world of energy, and they would write or speak about the scientific evidence for and experience of the subtle energies that provide our well-being.

Karagulla's *Breakthrough to Creativity,* for instance, describes many health professionals who daily use their subtle senses to help others heal. One example is a medical doctor who could tell exactly what was taking place in a patient's bodily organs and other systems as he examined them by palpating or other usual diagnostic procedures. He did have to run lab tests or do other conventional procedures in order to keep his license, but still, he just knew.

Karagulla also writes of Diane, a woman who had been clairvoyant from birth and who specialized in working with medical intuition. Karagulla enlisted Diane to sit in her waiting room and examine her patients with her insight as they waited to see the doctor. Diane was able to diagnose all of Karagulla's patients correctly. "Diane" was a pseudonym for my boss, Dora van Gelder Kunz. During my first years at the *American Theosophist,* one of my coeditors humorously said that working with Dora was like walking around with your psychic zipper down all the time. It was true. There wasn't an emotion or predisposition that you could hide from her. I have found the same to be true of Shannon.

Most of us, it seems, imagine ourselves to be alike in our perceptions of the world around us; we believe, aside from our own individual unique personalities, thoughts, and feelings, that we see the world in a more or less similar way. We agree that blue is blue, sulfur is odiferous, sandpaper is rough to the touch, lemon is sour to the taste, and the sound of a squeaking hinge on a door is irritating. But the perceptions of some of us are different.

When I was young, my mother told me a story illustrating the power of higher sensory perception. My father was a US Army Air Corps pilot during the Second World War. One midnight during the war, in Rockford, Illinois, my father's mother awoke from sleep and called out my father's name. She then said to my grandfather, whom her voice had awakened, "Something's happened to Ken." At that very same instant, my grandparents learned a few days later, the engine of my father's P-38 aircraft had failed as he was flying somewhere over the South Pacific. My father had radioed for help, but the plane was plummeting into the sea. The plexiglass canopy over the cockpit was jammed, and in order to get it open, my father had to kick at it repeatedly with all the strength he could muster so that he could parachute out of the plane. He eventually succeeded, but when the canopy came loose, it hit him in the head as it jettisoned off the aircraft. I assume it was at this time that my grandmother sensed his emergency. My father did manage to jump out of the aircraft, and later, US Navy personnel on a ship in the area found him and his parachute floating in the sea and ferried him to a hospital vessel.

There are countless such stories that could be told of precognitive knowing and intuitive insights. However, there are not many people such as Shannon who have such highly developed intuitive skills they are able to access on a daily basis. Their unusual experiences beg us to pause and open our minds a little more.

Shannon is an especially gifted healer. She has not only had supersensory perceptions and insights from an early age, she has also practiced and mastered her skills as she has matured, almost living in two worlds. You will see that she had unusual needs as a child. By the time she was six years old, she knew she could see things that most people could not but that were very important. However, she was punished and confined because of her outspoken revelations. Such a difficult childhood—one in which she had to go within her mind to cope—ultimately helped her to hone her supersensory perceptions and insights. I use the term *supersensory* to mean those senses beyond the five physical senses.

I always have a feeling of fun and delight when I work with Shannon, and I appreciate having been a part of bringing some of her experience and insight to others. I love reading case histories, and this book tells of just a few of thousands of Shannon's healing experiences. Readers will also be fascinated with some of the principles of healing she describes that anyone can put into use. They will meet a woman now in her eighth decade in life, someone who has had an unusually vast array of experiences in the healing arts. We hope you will enjoy these stories about the power of healing with energy medicine.

—Scott E. Miners

Preface

The purpose of this book is multifold, but its main focus is to show how healing can happen easily when we let go of resistance. The introduction starts with some personal self-disclosure, descriptions of intuitive insights, and background of my attraction toward the helping and healing professions. The subject of the book is healing and well-being of myself and others from a perspective of the very real effects of energy medicine and intent, as well as the role of intuitive insight in helping others heal. The scope of the book encompasses personal disclosures of my path that led to healing and intuitive insight, case histories, and bridges from science that corroborate the effectiveness of energy medicine and the fount of well-being from which it draws. In the epilogue, I have included many case histories that involve unusual healings as well as communications with those in the world of spirit. I think these healing stories will continue to become more common. Those that I have selected for this book are instructive, but they all give hope, no matter what the current physical condition might be. I include some disclosures about my life not only to highlight my own healings from various conditions, which hopefully will inspire others, but also so that the reader might gain more insight into how I do what I do and what inspires me to want to help others heal.

—Shannon McRae

Introduction

The Girl Who Could See What Others Could Not

God came to my house and asked for charity. And I fell on my knees and cried, "Beloved, what may I give?" "Just love," He said. "Just love."

—ST. FRANCIS OF ASSISI, in *Love Poems from God*

From an early age I knew things others did not know because, as it turns out, I could see things others could not see. I did not know at first that I was different from anyone else, but with the hindsight of a young adult it eventually became clear that what I was experiencing were unusual perceptive and intuitive insights. When I was a child I often had anxiety attacks in the middle of the night because I could sense beings in the room with me. So many nights I would pull the covers over my head in fear, my heart pounding, sometimes not ever returning to sleep. I have always described the beings I saw as very tall, silvery figures; Eben Alexander gave a similar description in his book *Proof of Heaven*, a story about his out-of-body experiences.

At first I did not know that I was having extrasensory insight, as I thought it was fairly normal—just as seeing and hearing are—for everyone to perceive the usually unseen or know it as I did. Perhaps my unusually difficult childhood, the aloneness and the long periods of turning inward, became a setting for the development of what has been called higher sensory perception. My childhood created a situation in which my inward life became more pronounced than for most people. Perhaps my intuitive abilities are also the result, as some believe, of soul experience. Whatever the reasons, because I was forced to go inward because of difficult outer circumstances, I began to notice I had insights and intuitions about people and things that just came into my mind easily and naturally.

A few key events serve as examples of how I was challenged by my childhood because of my strong sense of knowing; they also forced me to turn inward and gain even more refined insights. My whole experience as a child was centered mostly around my mother, father, grandfathers, and my pet dog, Fluffy, who was given to me when I was about two and a half years old. I had Fluffy, my very best friend and confidant, until I was eleven. She held all of my secrets, all of the heartfelt feelings I could not express to others, and every day I spent as much time with her as was allowed.

One of my earliest memories is of my grandfather coming for a visit by train when I was almost two. My mother left me with a Mrs. Vernon while she went to the train station to meet my grandfather. At one point I woke up from a nap and began asking for my mother to get me out of my crib, not unlike any other two-year-old might have done. Mrs. Vernon tried to calm me. She said that my mother was at the train station to meet my grandfather and would return soon. I somehow knew, however, that she was not at the station and cried out over and over, saying as best I could in a two-year-old's voice that she was not there. Mrs. Vernon had not deserved to be the focus of my screaming and sobbing, as she thought she was being kind and gentle, and she was. Later, Mrs. Vernon learned that my mother had actually been at the grocery store at the exact time I was told she was at the train station. Somehow I already knew that. Later in my life, my mother confirmed that this was true.

My earliest memory of feeling that I was different from other children was at the age of three. When my mother took me to be enrolled in a preschool across the street, I looked at all the kids there and thought, "How immature they all seem." I knew that I understood some things they did not. My mother asked me to go play with the other children as she talked with the teacher for a bit. I saw the children jumping around on the floor, playing with blocks and doing things children do. I went back to my mother and said, "I'm not going to play with them; they're little kids, and I'm not." I felt they were doing child's play and saw it as childish. I could not figure out why they were interested in such childish things. I told my mother that no, I would not go to that preschool. She knew when I said "no" in this way that I meant it, so she did not enroll me at all, knowing very well that I would otherwise start building up into a loud temper tantrum.

Another incident I remember is when I was almost four. I had a teddy bear doll I took everywhere, and I slept with it every night. One day my mother told me we were going to visit some of our friends, some relatively poor people, and that I was to bring my teddy bear doll. I objected because, since I carried it everywhere , I knew from her specific asking that I would never see my teddy bear doll again. While we were at the friends' house, their little girl began to play with my doll, and, seeing how delighted she was, my mother said I had to leave my teddy bear doll with the girl. I already knew ahead of time this was going to occur, and the hurt I felt inside was so deep that I could only sob, shaking with hurt and sadness as we drove home. It took many afternoon naptimes and nights before I could get to sleep easily again, and I never got a true explanation of why I had to give my beloved teddy bear away. In many ways, this incident set a pattern in my life in which I believed that I was not good enough to have things I loved.

When I was five, my family moved to another small town in California. My mother gave me a coloring book soon after, and I always colored outside the lines of people's bodies on the pages. My mother pointed out, "You are supposed to color inside the lines of the people's bodies." I rejoined, "But I see colors outside the lines of people when I look at them, and so I should color them like I see people." My mother, still not knowing what to think of these kinds of assertions from me, took an authoritative stance and threatened to take the coloring book away. I agreed to abide by the rules, but I hid the book under my bed and continued to color in my own way. (I later learned that the colors around people's bodies are called auras or bio-fields and that the colors signify certain frequencies of thought and emotion.)

A girl my age lived just up the street, and we played together at times. I was allowed to play with her because my mother trusted her mother and certainly had explained to her about my "strangeness." My mother was a confidential friend, and one day this woman confided that she was not able to have any more children. Later, even though I had not known about the contents of that conversation, I could see intuitively that she had become pregnant. I saw the soul of the new baby connected to the mother's energy. I knew it was going to be a boy. When I heard my mother say one day that the woman could not have any more children, I blurted out, "Oh, she's going to have a baby boy." I could not keep my mouth shut when I knew the truth. My mother was fit to be tied at yet another bald assertion from her child. She chastised me, called me a liar, and said, "How could you be so stupid to say such things?" I heard these sorts of comments a lot during the years I lived with my mother, but I knew what I knew. In fact, within eight months the woman gave birth to a baby boy.

Another example of things I just knew involved my step-grandmother, who was only a few years older than my mother. It was common knowledge in the family that my step-grandmother wanted to have a baby, but I intuitively sensed she would not be able to become pregnant. It was just something I knew, but my step-grandmother became hysterical when I told her, in my childish way, that she would never have a child of her own. My mother learned of my disclosure and again scolded me, saying, "Why can't you just keep your mouth shut."

Nevertheless, time came around to prove that I was correct, as my step-grandmother never did have a child. Years later she said that she had always felt very sorry for me and wished that I could have been her child. The love that poured through her to me may very well be why I lived through so many severe illnesses and why, even though it caused a family rift, I always felt blessed to have her in my life. In fact, she revealed to me that one day when I was about eleven, she was sitting in her rocking chair praying, as she did every afternoon. Suddenly, my paternal grandmother, who had passed away before I was born, came to her in a "vision," as she described it. She said that my grandmother asked her to pray for me every day, and she kept her promise to do so until the day she made her crossing.

Those were trying times for me as a young girl. As with all children, I was learning to observe the world around me and trying to make sense of it. I did many things any other child my age might, such as taking piano lessons when I was about seven. Sometimes I would hear my friends practicing in their own homes when I was outside playing or walking past, and I would call at the door and ask to come in. Every time I was invited in to listen and play the piano with my friends, my mother would soon call me to come home. Whenever my mother could not see me around in the house or just outside, she would call relentlessly for me because she was anxious; she worried because of the many times I had said something about someone that later came true, and she did not want people to think her daughter or herself strange. Because of her fear that I would say something that would embarrass the family, when I was six she instructed me not to go into her or my friends' homes any more, but I did not always follow her rules.

ILLNESSES, INSIGHTS, AND LIGHT AND SILVERY BEINGS

One more example of unfolding intuition came when I was six and a half. My mother and I were in the corner drug store. I saw a woman my mother knew who was pregnant, and I said to my mother in my loud, six-year-old voice, "Her baby is going to be born sick." My mother knew the lady; we lived in a very small town at the time, and, embarrassed for herself and me, she immediately whisked me out of the store. However, I was correct; a short time later the baby was born, became ill, and died within a few days. My mother told me, "Don't ever say anything like that again, because it came true," as if I had somehow caused the baby to die.

I was always a sickly child, and sometimes the illnesses were severe. When I was six I had rheumatic fever, which led to some remarkable experiences. The famous healer and medical intuitive Edgar Cayce also had rheumatic fever as a child. (I reflected on this many years later, when I had a fuller understanding of my involvement in healings for others and the intuitive insights I was, by then, used to receiving.) My bedroom was down the long hall at the front of the house. I was so ill with the rheumatic fever that I could hardly sit up in bed. I could not even look out the large picture window at the girls I heard playing in our front yard. I was also exposed to the measles and had a terrible time recovering from the effects. Those two illnesses played a role in developing my intuitive insight in order to help others heal, and they played right into my mother's desire to continue teaching me at home.

My mother was a teacher until I was born, and now she would come in to my room and teach me to read, particularly from assignments she had gotten from the school. I learned that she liked it when I was sick, not only to play out her desire to teach, but also because she could keep me separate from other kids; as I mentioned, she always worried that I would say things about what I saw that others could not see. She did not want word to get around the neighborhood that she had a strange daughter. Even when I was in school, she asked the teachers to keep me separate from the others, probably telling them I was prone to illnesses. My classmates would sit on a warm, thick rug on the floor during reading time, but I was made to wear horrid purple flannel pants my mother made for me and sit on a chair at the end of a row. I think this isolation was another reason I was sick so often and returned home to my bedroom for days at a time. It was psychologically difficult to be kept apart from others my age, and, looking back, I must have been very inept in socializing skills. I missed more school than I attended, but my mother achieved her goal of teaching me herself.

I had not only rheumatic fever followed by measles but also a number of other maladies; because I was so ill and isolated for so long, so alone, the fever and isolation served to take me to other realities. This period of time marked the beginning of a very unusual string of death experiences I had. Today the scientists call what I experienced "near-death experiences," or NDEs.

I had repeated NDEs. I knew at these times, as I experienced the dying process, that I could die for good, but I never did. One time, as my mother was driving me to a clinic, I had a strong feeling that I was needed here on earth. During that drive I experienced going through a tunnel to a light, and throughout this process I had many of the same thoughts and feelings described by others who have written about their NDEs. And just like so many of them, I was turned around by a loving being at the end of the tunnel and told I had to stay in my body and live this life because I had work to do. I said, "I don't want to work," but that was just my child mind reacting. This being also gave me the message that I would heal and survive.

One time I stayed at the clinic for four weeks, and a few years later I stayed for six weeks. Each time, I healed and gained weight at the clinic. Becoming ill, healing, and surviving became a theme in my life. Interestingly, my physician at the clinic was Francis M. Pottenger, Jr. This man is famous for his experiments with cats and is the author of *Pottenger's Cats,* a book that discusses the importance of nutrition in health not only for the individual, but also for future generations of children, as good health from sound nutritional practices by parents gets passed on through genes to children.

It was during this time period that I first saw the silvery figures in my room. These were very loving, spiritual beings. I saw them regularly after my second NDE, when I had been in the clinic for six weeks. Throughout my childhood I saw them during times of illness and the long times of being alone and quiet in my room. I saw these beings at least several times a week, if not every night. They appeared at dusk or in the middle of the night. The illnesses and long days and nights of isolation, with just my own conscious awareness of my feelings and subtle energies around me, became triggers to bring forward my desires to know more about life. I believe this is how my conscious awareness of the unseen parts of life developed.

The silvery figures were very tall, taller than most humans. They moved and shimmered. They seemed to be telling me that I needed to keep living. I see now, with the hindsight of experience, that they were telling me there was a reason to stay alive and grow up. These beings gave me a love and comfort I could feel that I did not get from my family, and this served to encourage me to stay and not go into the death experience. As I see it now, I know they were spiritual masters, unseen beings who often come to help all of us. Well, most people do not see them, but there are many who do, especially in childhood. Some people retain the ability as adults; with focus, anyone can sense unseen loved ones and helpers who are always with us. I have seen them all my life at various times, but the frequency of the visits changed after I turned eleven. They took on, or I perceived them in, a slightly different form, and sometimes even now, especially when the lights are off and my eyes are not being stimulated, I still see things like the silvery masters. They are just different in terms of their brightness; they are more like forms of energy.

I recall that I always felt very sad when my mother chastised me for things I said that she thought were imaginary, because I knew I was telling the truth. However, as I grew into adolescence, my sadness turned into anger whenever my mother did not believe me, and I would go into a rage of frustration. Nevertheless, as I matured I began to rely more on my own sense of self. In addition to the silvery masters, I also began to have extraordinary experiences of support from unexpected realms, even though I was still basically confined to my own home and room at this stage. I always felt safe and protected by these helpers in the spiritual realm and knew that I would come through all difficulties and be okay.

One example of the kinds of visits I had from those in spirit involved both of my grandmothers, each of whom died before my own birth in March of 1938. Even though they were gone, there were pictures of my grandmothers hanging on the walls in my home. I remember being quite sad that I did not have a grandmother; my friends all seemed to enjoy going to their grandmothers' homes, but I had not one to go to visit, and my step-grandmother was busy working at that time. I was home alone almost all the time, starting at age eight. I later learned a term that fit me then: I was a *latchkey* kid. My father, who was a geologist and chemical engineer, a miner, prospector, and researcher, worked full-time, and my mother always had committee meetings to go to during the day. During my alone time at home, when I was not so ill as to be confined to my bed, I often sat and gazed at the photographs of my grandmothers; one day I found myself wanting them to come alive so I could have the companionship of a true grandmother. The remarkable thing is that, in a unique way, they did come alive for me.

I remember being in front of the picture of my father's mother, talking to her in my mind, telling her I loved her and missed her and wanted her to come visit me. As I recall, she just sort of stepped out of the picture one day and then got bigger, expanding into a silvery, etheric body, then stood in front of me and smiled. I wasn't a bit afraid of this appearance because by now this kind of event was familiar to me. She talked to me about things like my dog and my love of trees and flowers and the sky. I "heard" her in my mind telepathically rather than verbally.

That incident was the beginning of my lifelong ability to see those who have died. It happens whenever I or someone I am talking with focuses on the deceased person. The person simply appears in front of me, just as my grandmother did. I have helped many people come to closure with loved ones who have passed over to the other side by communicating in this way. The people often appear to me with a message to give to their loved ones. No one really ever "dies," as in "ceases to be." The last chapter of this book addresses some of my experiences communicating with those who have passed away. This communication can be a very healing experience for people who are traumatized by the death of a loved one.

These childhood stories include just some of the early experiences I had, and they are examples of intuitive knowledge that comes to me, knowledge of things that one ordinarily would not know unless tuned in to one's inner guidance. These events were just the small beginnings of multitudinous experiences to come in the following years. As a child, I did not know that my intuitive knowing would serve me, as well as many others, in marvelous ways as my life unfolded. There were many challenges for me as a child and then as a teenager. My perceptions beyond the five senses were out of the ordinary. My assertions about my knowledge of (and to) others would continue to unsettle my mother the rest of her life and, therefore, my life with her.

SUMMARY

We all have pain and experience sorrow in varying degrees, depending upon our circumstances and our growth. My childhood experience, as painful as it was, opened me to a strong desire to find a way to communicate and understand the world. My family experience in general served to separate me from what is considered normal, but as I write my memories I see more clearly how I became hyper-psychic. In addition to isolation, the mixture of events that added to my development includes the pain of emotional and psychological abuses and being shipped away from home to health clinics for extended periods of time. I was also made to travel across the country alone to a school in my ninth grade, to a place where I knew no one, and then traveling alone again to return home.

Nevertheless, the richness of my inner life sustained me through many difficult circumstances like those. I learned to talk with a Master in the "inner world," and without such a strong desire to understand my outer world, I may not have met him. My mother had no interest in what I was experiencing, as I was a bother to her, but I found happiness by being with my friend, the Master, when I was desperate for companionship.

My high school years were quite painful because the other girls saw me as being too different to be a friend, so I was alone a lot then, too. During my junior and senior years I took solace, after eating and before the bell rang for afternoon classes, by reading a small *New Testament* and memorizing the words of Jesus, printed in red.

I remember also that I was an outcast with my in-laws, too. They would talk about me behind my back. I intuitively knew they were doing it. I later learned that they thought I was strange, and because of that and my hyper-intelligence (high IQ), they did not want me to fit in. I can see now, of course, where one could say that I was unusual because of my insights and behaviors, but at a young age I was super-sensitive and felt hurt by the ridicule and criticisms of others. I did not respond to reality the same as most people around me did, but then, I did not see reality the same as most. But I was just being myself.

When I would hear them whisper and speculate, I would "turn off" my hearing so I would not have to be aware of their comments.

However, turning off my awareness caused anxiety, as happens any time people shut off their sense of knowing. I did just know things, but they were things I could not tell anyone about because no one would believe me; I had to repress what I knew, and repression causes angst. I could be tipped off by the death of a relative far away, the news of a major accident, a freak weather pattern, or anything unusual. I was never aware of my behavior being strange; I was just being me, attuned to subtle information, as I had been all of my life.

I desperately wanted to know about myself. Why was I so different from everyone I knew? By this time I had had the experience of praying and intending healing for several people, and when healings did take place I was amazed. I remember, when I was about twenty, looking in the public library for a book that would help me understand myself and perhaps answer my questions about the healings. I saw the title *There Is a River,* by Thomas Sugrue, about the healer Edgar Cayce, and I immediately knew I had to read it. I learned about Cayce's life and how he was able to go into an altered state of consciousness and answer all kinds of questions from people everywhere about their health and their lives in general. Cayce knew things about people he had never met. I could relate. When asked, he would become quiet—just as I did in my alone times—and, lying on a sofa, he would give readings about the person who asked; he knew the person's physical health even when he or she was many hundreds of miles, even continents, away. His awareness seemed to transcend time and space and go into the microcosms within the body, and his readings and health advice helped thousands of people understand their lives and heal from very serious illnesses. This gave me great comfort and awareness because I thought, with what I knew, that I perhaps could help many people, too.

Through the ensuing years I studied and became proficient in anatomy and earned a doctorate degree in psychology. I do not work in the same way as Edgar Cayce did, as you will see, but I do know that what I do works for my clients. I hope some of the details in the chapters that follow will provide some insight and inspiration to readers about the well-being that supports us all.

1

Cellular Healing, Quantum Things, and Our Organizational DNA

> *Meditation—all by itself—may offer more to the health of [a person] than all the pharmaceutical remedies put together.*
>
> —**ROBERT DOZOR, *The Heart of Healing***

Energy medicine seems to work very well, and many case histories in the chapters that follow show how effective it can be. First, though, it is useful to lay a foundation as the basis of the most effective healings. Let us look at why so many have been healed outside the realm of conventional medicine's offerings of drugs and surgery. Why does energy medicine work so well? Why does spontaneous healing take place? These are questions that have multilayered answers, but our first clue is in what is said to be the smallest particles of our physical bodies, from which we have a viewpoint that can throw light on the answers. Thanks to scientific discoveries of the last century, the micro view of the human body is a remarkably effective perspective from which to consider the possibilities of healing that can take place far more easily than many have believed, because truly, our bodies are not as solid as they seem.

Let us look at quantum energy, which is the source for the physical body. Quantum physicists assert that a quantum is the tiniest amount of physical existence involved in interactions with other things. It is unusual to think of something smaller than molecules in your cells or genes in your DNA; even so, quantum energy plays a major role in the health of your body. Here I discuss how anyone can use this energy to change a physical illness by starting with cells anywhere in the body. This is what I do on a daily basis.

First we will look at some descriptions of this micro world as it relates to our bodies. Quanta are considered to be packets of matter with energy stored in them. Quantum physicists see quanta sometimes as waves, such as light waves—which are the building materials of our physical bodies—and sometimes as particles, such as photons; it depends on the way you observe them. Scientists argue that quanta alone can not only change their forms, but also do so when under human observation. This ability of the tiniest particles in our bodies to change form is important to remember in the context of intentional healing. In her book *The Quantum Self,* Dana Zohar refers to this phenomenon when she writes, "Something about the act of observation (or measurement) [changes] the quantum wave function"[1] of the energy being observed.

THE UNDERLYING ENERGY IN CELLS

Biophysicist Joyce Whiteley Hawkes attests to the energetic nature of the tiniest particles in the cells in our bodies. She describes the underlying reason that the intentional focusing of intent to heal is so effective: "Within each cell there are trillions of molecules composed of trillions more atoms. Like the spaces between stars, which contain huge amounts of energy, the ultrasmall nano-spaces inside of the atoms teem with energy to constantly manifest new creation."[2] It is actually at this ultra-small level that I do my healing visualizations, which involve building trillions of new, healthy cells in a microcosmic way; recent scientific observations give me the terminology to describe what I do. Let us look at how thought creates the quantum field that is at the basis for healing. To see how thought influences cells in the body, let us look at the highly sensitive cellular components in the context of thought.

Hawkes' description of the cellular environment is important to understand because it substantiates the workings of energy medicine at the micro level. For example, she avows, "In this microworld of the inner composition of your cells, energy and matter interface in ultrafast blips of time: nano- or pico-seconds. When an event occurs in these swift pulses of 10^{-9} or 10^{-12} seconds, the cells enter a type of quantum reality—no longer linear and no longer predictable."[3] We can create a non-linear (outside time) quantum field of healing reality through thought. I create this field through my thought when I am doing healing or practicing energy medicine (and you can too); I have been doing it as my profession for over forty years, so I am very practiced at it.

To do this, I create an intentional thought of healing, a field of healing, and work within it. When I generate a field of healing, it involves every part of the body, from the tiniest to the largest parts. Once I have created the healing thought field, I begin visualizing new, healthy cell regeneration. You can be assured that this energetic imprint is having an effect on the cells, which, at the building-block level, is not confined to linear time or space. Hawkes' scientific findings, as one example, point to this ability of cells to respond to any thought/quantum field. She writes, "The cell is the interface between ordinary and nonordinary reality; possibilities exist here that we have barely begun to understand or develop. . . . Yet we can influence them with our consciousness."[4]

Why does this kind of energy healing work? Quantum physicists have proved that human observation has an effect on the tiniest of things. Physicist Amit Goswami refers to the effect of our observation in this way: "Quantum physics in the form of its famous observer effect (how an observer's looking transforms quantum possibilities into actual experiences in the observer's consciousness) is forcing us to a paradigm shift from a primacy-of-matter paradigm to a primacy-of-consciousness paradigm."[5] It is especially clear to me that consciousness is primary. I do my work at this tiniest of energetic levels as well as with the whole system of the body, thoughts, emotions, and their fields. All of my clients who can align consciously with this kind of healing have had remarkable results.

Scientists need laboratory equipment such as electron microscopes to view subatomic particles, but I can see these tiniest of cellular particles in my intuitive perception. I can say that it truly is as if this quantum energy in our cells has a consciousness and responds to the observer. Goswami asserts that we have to look at the observer effect, "how our measurement or observation changes . . . possibility into actuality."[6] Knowing this, it is even more important to monitor our own thoughts and emotional energy—our attitudes—because we each observe the world continuously such that our bodies, our cells, and our DNA and genes can carefully align with healthy thought. It is advisable to think the best of all we observe. Our observations and thoughts change possibilities into actualities. The healthy, overall consciousness of well-being, or Source energy, is always there, ever possible to draw from, but we have to align with it, allow it, and stop resisting it in order to consistently have the flow of complete health. Basically, we have to think more like Source and refrain from judging anything or anyone, including ourselves.

Thought is an epigenetic factor that affects DNA, so it is important to align your thought to well-being (feeling good). (Throughout this book, I refer to *well-being* as meaning "Source energy," which is the basis of all life in the universe.) It is necessary to make observations of a positive nature in order to feel good. There was a Beach Boys song in the 1960s about good vibrations, and now it is known through science that thoughts create vibrations in the body and field. Pure thoughts such as unconditional love and appreciation are of high vibratory frequency. Being in love makes you feel high. Negative thoughts, such as judgment, shame, anger, and criticism, are lower vibratory energies. Our DNA interacts with thought and, to a certain extent, is negatively affected, compromised, or loses energy in the context of negative thinking. Chronic negative thinking leads to illnesses.

In healing work of any kind, it is important to remember that the cells are based in light, are made of light waves, and are therefore always in flux, always affected by the vibrations of the fields made with thought and feeling, and thus cells can be replicated in a healthy way. Examples of positive observations that align with the flow of well-being and healthy energy for our cells are: "My body is an extension of well-being, and my cells can vibrate as a match to well-being when I relax and allow the flow; I allow this vibration; I feel this vibration; I surrender to this vibration of well-being no matter where I am or what I am doing; I cease thinking any thought or doing any action that causes a feeling other than well-being; I forgive myself when I catch myself thinking negative thoughts; I observe myself as an extension of Source and feel the vibration of well-being in all my cells. I surrender and relax, trusting in my intuition and always aiming to choose the path that makes me feel good, positive, and loved."

OBSERVATIONS, SURRENDER, AND FIELDS OF HEALING ENERGY

My perspective in intuitive medicine and healing work is that the DNA in our cells are three-dimensional outposts for information from the overall field of well-being. DNA interacts with other multidimensional fields, including the many different thoughts and feelings that either block or harmonize with the natural flow of well-being energy. Incidents, self-criticism, and judgments that have not been forgiven become blockages to the flow of well-being. A negative thought creates a field that then feeds information to the DNA, which is listening to every thought. Thinkers—you and I—create energies from thoughts; we create what might have been merely a passing possibility into reality in our DNA and cells by our focused and repeated thoughts. You just have to practice thoughts that feel good and let go of all those that do not in order to serve the health of your body; by practicing with consistency, even unwanted conditions that have been with you a long time will disappear.

Let us look more at how the ultra-small DNA can respond to possibilities of healing and can positively affect our cells. Recent scientific findings indicate that our DNA organizes light waves,[7] the very light waves that quantum physics show us are changed by our observation. It can be said that DNA is listening to each thought for its instructions and organizing light waves in accordance; the finding that DNA organizes light waves into various patterns is another example of how DNA uses energetic information such as our thoughts and attitudes to replicate our cells in healthy or unhealthy ways. This fact of the power of thoughts and attitudes helps explain the stories of cancer cures, remissions, and healing of other diseases that defy conventional medical explanation. Individuals let go of their stressful thoughts and emotions, and heal.

Unmanaged stress negatively affects the DNA, adversely affecting the way it organizes the light waves that play such a central role in cellular replication, whereas peace positively affects DNA. Being peaceful and simple, appreciating the moment, stopping judgment, and being happy in the ever-present now all support the precise replication of healthy cells. The positive vibration of well-being is in the ever-present now, and since this positive vibration is the collective and individual source field of all that is (which I think is the same as the unified field described by Einstein), all you need to do is stop resisting it with all those stressful, negative thoughts. Meditation, rest, relaxation, movement, being at ease, and finding something to appreciate—nature, flowers, birds, the sky, the sun, bodies of water, and anything about anyone around you—all help immeasurably to redirect the flow of negative thinking.

As quantum science has shown, by observing what you want to change, you affect it. So let us look at how this might work in a healing interaction. The healing exchange between the healer and the client involves surrender to the possibilities of complete health. Through consciousness and intent, I (or any healer) can create a new individual field, a quantum possibility, by intending to help someone change a disease condition. This can be as simple as, for example, seeing what the healthy condition was intended to be prior to the condition of disease (which is the piling of cells in the body that occurs in a disease process). The diseased cells are not the same as the original healthy DNA blueprint. They have been altered by either stress or circumstances such as limited belief systems, judgments, and negative thinking in general. For example, suppose a person had been told something might occur to her because a parent had a certain condition. The consistent thought of the negative condition actually energizes the non-preferred condition. DNA has many possibilities. As people, each of us has unlimited choices about what we think, but we must focus on what we want and limit thoughts about what we do not want in order to stay aligned as much as possible with the flow of well-being. Even identical twins have unique health profiles, and research is showing this is because of epigenetic factors such as attitudes and lifestyle as well as the fact that DNA is multidimensional.

It is important to look at all these things in healing. I perceive multidimensional levels of reality. I close my eyes during the healing process because it helps me focus and see the organizing light coming from the healing fields that are fed by and provide well-being. Visualizing in this way helps me to co-create with my client a specifically intended and individual healing field that encompasses and adds energy to my client. This creates a field of intentional consciousness, where healing takes place with more energy. It places the client, and thus all the client's cells, in a space of quantum reality, where time and space do not exist. It is true, as Hawkes writes, that "the cells enter a type of quantum reality—no longer linear and no longer predictable."[8]

The possibility and probability of healing become reality when intent, belief, and desire are all in harmony for the healing to occur. A healing reality space occurs for me, too, when I am working. When I am on the phone with clients, I am only aware of them and the healing space around them. I am not aware of anything in the physical room around me. This is how I have come to understand what scientists call the quantum field of possibility. As I work, my clients feel different things: a sense of uplifting, a tingling, a lightness of being.

This is the best way I can describe the feelings that come from the field of the benevolent healing space that we create with our mutual intent for the client to be healed.

ENTERING A HEALING REALITY

If you have been blocking well-being by your stress or negative thoughts, you have to enter a different reality in consciousness to go into the healing space. You could call this space a vortex where well-being always exists. It is always there, it always provides health, and it is in all the dimensions of our DNA. You can change any physical condition. When I enter the healing space for a session, my words get garbled because I am in a different reality where words are not so useful or necessary. Conversation with clients during a healing session is not necessarily helpful, because if a client speaks while I am working, answering can sometimes take me out of the healing field, so I prefer the silent presence of clients. Working on the phone allows me to be more focused in that healing space.

Because every one of my clients has given permission for healing, not only are they open to the field of healing energy we create through thought, but also the degree of openness to the vortex of well-being, which is always there to feed us, is greater. Clients stop resisting the flow, and then it naturally becomes a stronger force. Because clients have asked for energy healing to be used, they are able to surrender to the healing process, which gains them entry into the special focus of healing space we co-create—which in turn helps facilitate the healing from the overall field. Their entry to the healing space shifts everything. It is as if the healer's intent along with the client's adds force to the well-being from the many dimensions that exist within and outside of our cellular DNA.

FORGIVENESS POWER

It is important for individuals to work to change the patterns of thought, emotion, or habit that keep their fields from being open to the ongoing healing energies of life. One of the main blockages, if not the central one, results from an event in which the other person has not been forgiven. This event could be anything from a moment of road rage to guilt or anger toward a parent or loved one. It is important to continually forgive, first yourself, and then others. You could say, "Okay, despite the fact that I got angry at that driver, I forgive myself and the other." It is so important to forgive. You could also say, "Okay, perhaps that person did not see me or is late and under stress; I forgive him. Wow! I realize I actually also need to forgive myself for immediately judging him." If you do not forgive and let go of such things on a daily basis, you will have blockages of emotional energy that can turn into physical blockages in your cells. Remember, DNA changes as a result of a negative thought or experience; the way I see it, the DNA loses some of its light energy.

One of the first things I ask my clients to do in forgiveness work is to make a list of all the thoughts and feelings of a negative nature over the entirety of their lives, from shame and guilt to anger and anxiety, and to forgive themselves. This releases blockages from the psyche and, in turn, allows the cells of the body to fully function in well-being. You do not need to go back in time and hunt everything down, but if a memory surfaces, whether from earlier in the day or earlier in your life, and it is a judgment of yourself, you can just forgive yourself right then.

Our bodies store light, our DNA organizes it, and we align with its natural beauty by our thoughts and emotions. We dim the light when we have not forgiven ourselves and others or when we have thoughts of judgment or negativity. Forgiveness puts you back in your power, so when you ask someone else for assistance and you are asking from the power of well-being that is naturally in you and is loving and good to you and all others, you are not asking from a place of weakness.

QUANTUM PACKETS OF ENERGY

When I work with the intent to heal, it could be said that I use quanta, little packets of energy, to help the healing process. I help to release packets of energy from cells that are dysfunctional, cells that are piling up in heaps from negative energy and have been changed from their original positive, healthy energy. These damaged cells are often the result of continuous negative observations, as might be described by quantum physics. They can be further brushed off by such visualizations as the image I use of being scrubbed away, as if the cells are little tiny soap bubbles on the kitchen counter. The intention and focus is what helps make possible this transfer of old cells out of the body and into the field around it to be eliminated.

At the same time I see the clumps of unhealthy cells and scrub them away, I also, as though I have an airbrush, paint new, pristine, original, healthy blueprint cells. I see these cells as flowing through the brush by the trillions from the Source field of well-being. These cells contain original, healthy, multidimensional DNA. This process causes new cells to replicate and replace the old, unhealthy cells. I imagine the old cells to be leaving the body, the field. Remember that observation has a powerful effect on physical systems. I know that this process works at the level of DNA and cellular repair. Before I start to work, I tell my clients that they might feel warmth, tingling, or something different. About seventy-five percent of my clients say they feel the changes, but even for those who do not, the healing is still working.

Another way to say this is that the quantum well-being field that underlies DNA has within it the source coding for original, healthy DNA. Despite the epigenetic factors such as negative thinking or environmental toxins that may have caused compromised cellular DNA to create unhealthy cells, new, healthy DNA can be generated by intent aligned with this quantum field. Then this new yet original DNA creates from within the cell nucleus new, healthy cells to replace those that are diseased. As you read the case histories in the rest of this book, just imagine this taking place with many of those who experienced healing.

SELF TALK FOR CELLS

Dawson Church, author of the remarkable book *The Genie in Your Genes,* writes,

> The use of visualizations to help patients cope with cancer was pioneered by Carl Simonton and others in the 1970s. I vividly remember an interview I did with a woman in 1989. She impressed me as someone with great strength of will and courage.
>
> Nancy had been diagnosed with metastasized Stage IV uterine cancer in 1972. Though her condition was terminal, she had rejected conventional medical therapy entirely, reasoning, "My body created this condition, so it has the power to uncreate it too!" She quit work, exercised as much as her physical energy allowed, and spent hours lying in the bath. She came up with a visualization that tiny stars were coursing through her body. Whenever the sharp edge of a star touched a cancer cell, she imagined it puncturing the cancer cell, and the cancer cell deflating like a balloon. She imagined the water washing away the remains of the dying

> cancer cells. She focused on what she ate, how far she could walk, her baths, and the stars.[9]

Church describes what happened next:

> Nancy began to feel stronger, and her walks became longer. She began to visualize what her future might look like many years from that time. She went back to see her doctor three months after the diagnosis. She did not make the appointment until she had a firm inner conviction that the cancer was completely gone. To the astonishment of her physicians, tests revealed her to be cancer-free. Curiously, many patients who use similar techniques report an inner knowing that the disease is gone, long before it is confirmed by medical tests. They also use highly individualized images that work for their particular psyche.[10]

So, just as in Nancy's case, you can tell your subconscious to listen to your soul, which is connected to well-being. In a way, this intelligence in the soul is what talks to the body and tells it to produce original-blueprint, healthy cells. You can also visualize an audience of DNA with genes on their laps sitting and listening to you. Talk to them, and tell them how much you love them and how wonderful they are for replicating cells precisely. You can tell the gene in charge of cellular replication to re-energize and replicate cells just as in the original, healthy blueprint. Allow yourself to be full of the energy that well-being provides, and feel it as it livens and refreshes your body. As I understand more of this work today, I am aware that, in a sense, I become a subset of a client's unseen DNA; I become one with it. I see the complete health of each person residing in this unseen energy that feeds our DNA. This total health can be part of anyone's life at any time.

It is good to practice bringing yourself into a feeling state of compassion. This will allow you to feel the connection that brings us all together. The reason many people can feel the energy of change in their cells when I work with them is partly because of our mutual intention, but it is also because of the collective quantum field of well-being that supports the change desired. When working as a healer, either for yourself or another, you just hold the space and listen; when you are devoid of judgment, separation cannot be seen. Others will be able to feel this and stay present in this healing space. That is where the benevolence of healing comes in: there is benevolence, and all you have to do is allow it.

2

Healing an Arterial Tear, Genetic Potential, and Removing Cancer Cells

> ***What is intuition? Why do you call certain thoughts intuition? Because there is no rational explanation for such thoughts; there is no contextual precedent for such thoughts. An intuition is your glimpse at a quantum leap.***
>
> —**AMIT GOSWAMI,** *Quantum Activism*

The diversity of clients I have worked with requires me to provide a number of different services. I have for a long time, therefore, integrated my work as a medical intuitive and energy medicine health professional with my practice as a psychologist, and in the last fifteen years as a nutritionist, as well. There are many examples I could give of the diverse needs my clients have presented, but here I want to focus on two client cases that demonstrate how subtle energy healing can take place in several different ways. This is a kind of healing that might seem unusual to some, but to me it is quite natural. (Throughout the book, all client names are pseudonyms to protect their privacy.)

Recently, Grace telephoned about her husband, Larry, whom she said wanted immediate help. She was in the ER with him. She said that at first Larry had a nosebleed that would not stop, so they went to the ER, where the doctor put cotton tubes up his nose to soak up the blood and stop the flow. However, blood then started coming from Larry's eyes. The staff at the ER called an ear, nose, and throat physician, who attempted to stop the bleeding by cauterizing the area inside Larry's nose.

Because Grace asked me to help, I was focusing on Larry and receiving impressions about him while she talked. I immediately knew the nose and septum were not the cause of the problem. I said to Grace as gently as I could, because she was already upset, "I think I see an aneurysm that has occurred in Larry's brain." I also told her I thought it was serious. In fact, I knew it was.

Although I knew it was an aneurysm, I did not want to say that so strongly or directly because I did not want to scare Grace, who was extremely distraught. So I softened my comment to, "I think I see. . . ." I also intuitively knew the doctors were not going to do a brain scan and therefore would not discover the aneurysm. Thus, I felt that I had to help heal it, which is essentially what Grace requested on Larry's behalf.

HEALING PROCESS

Now I am going to describe in more detail what happens for me when I am focused on a client and therefore focused on the healing flow to assist them. This healing process brings to me an immediate awareness of the client's condition. For example, in Larry's case I immediately became aware of a bulge in an artery, which I saw may have been an aneurysm, in his frontal brain. A tiny arterial tear about one-sixteenth-inch long had occurred in it. It is hard to describe how awareness of such conditions comes to me; however, I know my focus involves a strong desire to help someone, and I think it is because of this desire that I am pulled into an awareness of what is taking place within someone's body. I have a seminal wondering of what is going on that takes just an instant, and then I find myself seeing, in complete reality, whatever the condition is. It seems the intention to help someone acts as a powerful attracting force. I feel myself pulled right to the main problem by some unseen but benevolent force as soon as I intend to help and question what is taking place.

When I begin to help someone by identifying his or her condition and helping them heal, whether physical or emotional ills, it is as though I am given access to a unified field of information that goes beyond a client's individuality. The feeling I have is one of knowing that I am a part of what I am observing. It might help to look more at this process using Larry's case as an example.

Initially, when Grace first telephoned, I used the power of visualization of anatomy to follow the path of the bleeding she described up through the septum so that I could see what was happening. As I focused on doing this for just an instant, I was immediately pulled to the source of the problem, and perceived the stark fact that there was a tear in an artery in his brain. I knew this was not an issue with the sinuses, septum, or nasal passage; problems in these areas were only outcomes of the bleeding from the tear.

Blood redirected to Larry's eyes after the doctor plugged his nose. As I began working to heal this tear, I was fully present with my awareness, just as in all my healing cases.

It is hard to put this in words, but when I am healing, it is like being present in a much larger consciousness that encompasses me as well as the person I am helping. Some greater force brings me into alignment in this way.

There is an immediate and palpable sense of being pulled to awareness of conditions that enables me to help others to heal; in Larry's case, as soon as I wished to help, I was somehow next to the tear, seeing it as if I was about the same size as it. From this vantage point I worked to close the tear by energetically pulling in trillions of healthy cells to mend it. Helping pull these cells together takes a lot of focus. You could call it visualizing, but it is just a bit more than that, since I actually see them coming together as an outcome of intent.

I feel as though I am aligned with a much greater intelligence within a consciousness that sources cells, and this consciousness feeds on intention and focus. In Larry's case, I grabbed bunches of cells that just appeared from the unified field during the healing process. I wrapped the area around the tear with all these new cells, trillions of them. They then formed a sort of bandage that helped repair Larry's artery. The bleeding stopped, though the doctors thought it was something they had done. A month later, Larry was doing well.

Work of this nature takes very intense focus, and while I am focusing, it is as if nothing else in the world exists. This work is so engaging, so graphic, that I sometimes actually feel a gag response as I am working, which is interesting, because I have a very high tolerance to almost anything having to do with the physical body. I did hands-on hospice work for many years, and I saw just about everything during that time. But this work of intuitive healing brings me so close to the functions of the body that staying balanced can be challenging.

My experience helps me know what to do in healing many different types of conditions, from emergencies to even the most minor problems. As in Larry's case, my knowledge of cellular structure gives me confidence in what I am doing. I have seen wounds heal before, so when I am working, I am thinking positively that healing will take place. I also know from the feelings I have and the level of awareness this work takes me to that there are unseen forces at work.

These include the client's intention, which I cannot interfere with, as well as my own healing intent and the influence of benign forces in the overall unified field.

WHAT CAUSES DIS-EASE?

It is true that potentially any dis-ease in the physical body that is not caused by an incident such as an accident can occur for anyone. But well-being is always the greatest potential. One must focus on this with a positive attitude to support health, even in the face of unwanted conditions. Even when you are in pain you can have hope instead of fear. It is a fine line between being positive and being fearful.

Stress is centrally involved in illness and dis-ease. For example, many of my clients have said that they feared they would inherit a condition from a parent. To think we are genetically preset for dis-ease is a fearful and incorrect thought. Our genes have many potentials, and they are very affected by lifestyle and environmental factors, such as stress, positive thinking, and healthy food choices.

Differing levels of stress occur for each person, depending upon the extent of the person's fear. How often does one replay a fearful thought? What happens when one keeps thinking the same thought? Belief forms! Another way to describe the basis of dis-ease is to discuss the resonance of thought and emotion.

For example, someone who is fairly focused on fear of a certain dis-ease condition occurring will simply draw more of those thoughts into his or her own mind. It is like the vibration of a guitar string: When you pluck a string, it vibrates with forms of wave energy. The string next to it will vibrate more subtly, but nevertheless will form similar wave harmonics. Focusing on any particular thought creates waves of energy that not only affect the strings of energy in particles in the body, but also in the fields of energy around us. The law of harmonic attraction provides more thoughts like the one a person keeps thinking. So, if people continually think of what they fear, more thoughts and emotions of what they fear will manifest even more strongly. Even if people just imagine they feel some condition they do not want, the imagination attracts more of the same kind of thought and emotional energy.

The way out of negative thinking about anything—and specifically, this example of fear of genetic predisposition to dis-ease—is simple. Start by realizing and feeling that the predominant basis of life is well-being. It is important to focus on the well-being you do have in your life as well as all the well-being that has been part of your ancestry, and to completely stop thinking you are genetically predisposed to illness. Your genes are programmed with all potential and holographic memory of the human genetic code, so it is important to focus on what you want, such as the well-being that is at the basis of all life.

This mind-body-emotion scenario is similar in principle to all the many other kinds of cases I work with. For example, one of my clients, Barbara, called saying she had cancer in her left breast and wanted my help to heal it. Even though she gave me her diagnosis, I asked for her permission to scan her body intuitively. As usual, as I scanned I used my awareness to perceive what was going on inside her body. When I see something that is out of order—such as, in this case, a swollen lymph node in the left armpit—it is as if I shrink down and change perspective so that I am right next to the thing. This may sound strange, but somehow I am able to be aware within a person's body. Then I can see what is taking place, even at the cellular level. It is so vivid and real to me.

With Barbara's aligned intent, I started to get rid of the darker cells by sweeping them away. Cancer cells appear to me as sick, dark cells, and as I pull these cells away, I simultaneously replace them with healthy cells. Sometimes I use an imaginary vacuum cleaner. I suggested to one client that she use an imaginary little helper who vacuumed out the cells as I worked. She even named her imaginary helper. As the vacuuming process takes place, I focus on pulling in new cells. I visualize my hands being just a bit larger than the cells themselves, and I visualize layering on new cells. Because of this focus, the cells are being manufactured according to intent, just as I described in Larry's case. The cells arise from the energy field of both my desire and the client's; some clients have strong intention, and the stronger it is, the more this alignment helps. This reminds me of the seminal work of Carl Simonton, who, many years ago, developed a method of visualization that helped clients reverse illnesses. Many people do not use enough focus or confidence in their intention and their ability to create, but they do want to heal, and this is enough to allow someone such as myself, with intention, to help bring the healing.

As this process takes place, I observe whether the new cells continue to hold their original DNA blueprint of complete health. Whether the new, healthy cells hold or whether dark, sick cells start to grow back depends on many factors: how the person thinks, feels, and eats; stress levels; and relationships. People often need to reevaluate many things in their lives, including limiting beliefs, in order to heal. Often, follow-up sessions are necessary in order to address these issues.

REMINDERS AND CHANGES

Many people require coaching to realign with healthy thoughts. Remembering to focus on health rather than illness takes constant monitoring of one's thoughts. Also, it is important to examine negative habits and lifestyle factors such as poor food choices. You need commitment to your health if you want to be healthy.

3

Healing Cells and Repairing an Eardrum

What a piece of work is man! How noble in reason! How infinite in faculties! In form and moving, how express and admirable! In action, how like an angel! In apprehension, how like a god! The beauty of the world! The paragon of animals!

—Hamlet, 2.2.250

I offer the thoughts and experiences in the case histories in this book to all readers who may want assistance in healing of any kind or who would like to use the information as learning material to help others heal. Certainly the way I use my abilities, what I do, is unique to me, but it is just as certain that anyone with the intent and focus to heal or help others to heal may do so, as well.

Through intuition, we can so align with someone else who makes the request in body, mind, and emotions that we can know, often more than the person himself or herself knows, what is taking place energetically, whether at the cellular level or in thought and emotion. Why? It is because we are not really separate at the basic dimension of our lives. Science is proving more and more that everything in the universe is connected and exists in many dimensions. Quantum physicists have made huge strides in finding out how these connections work, and this science has also helped me to understand more concretely what I do with intuitive healing. A key to the ability to heal is that nothing, including the physical body, is solid; scientists have proven this through their study of particle physics.

Many of us realize that we can communicate by extrasensory perception, and scientific testing has proven this ability beyond dispute. For example, we have known for years about the secret psychic training in the former USSR and the United States, in which psychics worked with their governments to try to change the thoughts of targeted individuals. These psychics were also trained in a technique called "remote viewing," meaning that they could travel through space and time to view places and things to help their countries move forward in their quests. Today there are classes in many countries that teach these techniques, and police departments nationwide have used the services of remote viewers.

Many of us have been given what might be described as gifts, and one might call mine the gift of being able to align with another person on the physical, emotional, and cellular levels and understand the blockages to complete health. You could call this a form of remote viewing. I am not a spy, however, nor would I ever invade another's privacy, and I only use my intuitive viewing when a client requests it of me. I will say more about the kinds of insights I experience and how they help me help others in the case histories in this and the following chapters, but first I wish to address a few basic concepts.

We know that our thoughts and emotions affect our physical bodies in many different ways. Stress plays a prime role in the creation of dis-ease, and it can come from memories of the past—buried memories that have not surfaced—and fears, anxieties, and worries. Our thoughts and emotions are so powerful, as witnessed millions of times in people's lives, that it behooves each of us to monitor where they take us and consider how they affect our well-being.

There is power in thoughts and emotions. Many people are becoming more aware of how they can affect our bodies and, perhaps, the physical bodies of others. This was a novelty thought for me until I started noticing how I felt around others. Those who had a positive outlook on life felt lighter, and I felt uplifted around them; when I was near those who were depressed, angry, or without hope, I noticed a heavy feeling. I realized as I matured that I could control my own personal environment with an ongoing positive attitude and outlook on life.

Even though much of what I know and the way in which I work with clients have to do with seeing thoughts and emotions that have led to dis-ease, I have also long had an ability to perceive where a dis-ease is occurring in the body's cells. I can see where a stress in a person's life, whether from thought, emotion, or environmental reasons, has caused the body to need repair. Regarding this healing at the cellular level, I can say that when a client requests my help in this way, I can use remote viewing to view through the cells, through the mitochondria (the energy centers of the cells), and on to the place of nothing but pure white light, where all cells are connected on all levels. From this perspective I see the dis-ease that might be present, the cause of the dis-ease, and the way to heal it.

APPEARANCE OF CANCER CELLS

A good example of what I see at the physical level and how I work with the cells themselves occurs with cancer cells, which do not die; they just pile up on each other. Cancer cells do not appear alive and brilliant to me as healthy ones do. Healthy cells sparkle and bubble; cancer cells do not have this brilliance. They are not following the pattern of the cellular processes of dying and replacing themselves.

Cancer cells appear sludgy because they are not going through the process of normal replicating and dying. When I first scan, I see a dark area when there is cancer growing, whether it is in the skin, the bones, or an organ. When I then focus on the particular area, I see the sludgy-looking cancer cells themselves. When I start getting the visual of the cancer, such as when I work directly with people in hospice situations, I also receive an olfactory signal, what I call an "odor of cancer." I have been experiencing these impressions for more than forty years.

PATCHING A HOLE IN AN EARDRUM

I discuss several cases of cancer in later chapters, but following is one example from thousands of cases I have experienced when someone called asking for a healing for a friend. It illustrates how I use remote viewing as well as the power of virtual healing when a client's intent is an essential part of the healing process.

A woman from Arizona called me one day and asked if I could help her male friend. Tom was in Montana and would be traveling in the next few days to Oregon, Northern California, and back to Arizona, as he was a truck driver. I replied that I would be willing to try to help him, so she and I arranged a time for me to call him on his mobile phone while he was on the road.

When I called, Tom told me that he had a punctured eardrum from a recent scuba diving experience. He had been to his doctor and had taken antibiotics for over a month, and yet he was still experiencing pus oozing from the puncture and was developing a small rash below his ear. Of course, I became quite alarmed, yet I knew intuitively that I might be able to help him, at least somewhat. To begin, I made the suggestion that he might want to visit an emergency room if his eardrum felt worse.

Tom agreed with me, though he wanted immediate help from me using energetic medicine, as he was on the road driving his truck for the next few days. I started working with him and began the healing process by "seeing" the eardrum itself. As I looked at it from the inside, I could see where the pus was forming. I virtually pulled the pus away from the site by using the energies of healing intention and seeing a healing take place; then, in the same way, I put a patch made of millions of cells on the eardrum to seal up the leakage. I also cleansed the area, as I was very aware of what the infection would do. His ear doctor had told him that he had a strep infection, but I intuitively felt it was staph. I continued to work with him until I felt we were complete for that time.

Two days later, still on the road, Tom called from Northern California and said that his eardrum felt better, the pus flow had decreased, and the rash had diminished. I had been thinking of him often after our session, as I usually do with my clients, sending healing energy. He said he could tell when I was thinking about him and sending the healing energy, as he felt peace and calmness during those times. During this second call I continued the process of healing his eardrum by energetically cleansing and healing the entire area, inside and outside, and I could see a definite improvement.

Three days later I received another call from Tom, saying he had made it to Arizona, the eardrum felt even better, the pus was gone, and the rash had completely disappeared. He said he had an appointment with his ear doctor in a few days, thanked me for what I had done to help in the healing process, and said he could still tell when I was thinking about him.

About three weeks later we had our next phone call. Tom shouted into the phone, "Dr. McRae! I'm so happy to hear your voice! Do I have a story for you!" I was, of course, delighted to hear his enthusiasm and listened as he continued. "I went to my ear doctor, as I said I would, and as he was looking in my ear and at my eardrum, he said, 'Hmm, this is strange.' We both looked at the Q-tip he had had in my ear, and he said, 'This looks like a little patch of skin or something.' I started laughing, because he wouldn't have believed me if I had told him you put a patch there, but he did say the eardrum had healed and the hole wasn't there anymore." Then he and I shared our mutual delight about the experience, and I told him his would be one case I wouldn't forget.

Tom had had an emergency, and because of it, he was very focused and intent upon healing. He believed in energy medicine and in my abilities, and a healing took place. It is important to reiterate that it is not just my own intent and virtual skills that are involved; the energy and intent of the person desiring healing is also needed. Wherever two or more are gathered for the same purpose, the power is amplified beyond measure. This is the case with all of the healings I describe in the following chapters.

4

Presence, Prayer, and Healing a Headache

> ***For most of our existence as a species, we have not had doctors, whether conventional, alternative, or otherwise. The survival of the species alone implies the existence of a healing system.***
>
> —**ANDREW WEIL**, ***Spontaneous Healing***

I mentioned this in the introduction to this book but will repeat it here: As a result of a very difficult set of circumstances throughout my early childhood, including many illnesses, I turned far inward, to my inner self, where I learned remarkable things. In fact, I went so far in my alone times, which were constant, that I began to have what I now know were very deep and unusual insights and experiences. Most of those experiences were prescient beyond the five senses.

As a girl, I naïvely disclosed my intuitions to those around me and was punished for what I thought was normal insight, and as a result, my childhood became very difficult. But I knew what I knew, and I saw the outcome of what I could often sense was going to happen in the people around me, whether it was a sickness that manifested or a condition that reversed itself.

PAIN CAN LEAD TO EMPATHY

Now, several decades later, many times each day in my work in intuitive medicine, I am inspired to reflect and meditate and to give thanks for the gifts that I have. I attribute my ability to "tune in" and perceive illnesses and physical and emotional challenges in others to my profound need to understand what was going on during the difficult times of my childhood. The pain I experienced then definitely helped me to be empathic. As a result of my experiences in knowing the unseen that was occurring in people's lives when I was a child, I began to realize that I could use this gift to help in healing work. As a young adult, I made a vow to use my active extrasensory abilities to help others, and I have been doing so for close to fifty years now. Over the years I have not only honed these intuitive abilities, but I have also undertaken extensive academic training in the helping professions, including nutrition and many informal and extracurricular trainings.

The first time I was asked to help heal someone was when I was about twenty-five years old. A woman at my church who knew a little about my background asked me to pray for a friend of hers. I immediately closed my eyes, went into the silence that was so familiar to me, and asked in the name of All That Is for this woman to be healed of her affliction. I perceived what was going on with her and felt myself being a conduit for healing energies consciously flowing to heal her condition. I later learned from her friend that she had improved tremendously within days. It made me think again of the bible phrase, "For where *two* or three *are gathered* together in my name, there am I in the midst of them,"[1] or, therein is complete healing if desired by the two or more who are doing the asking.

PRAYER, COMPLETE HEALTH, AND THE UNSEEN

My clients now routinely ask me to intuitively scan their bodies and their emotions, the latter of which can cause physical difficulties if unresolved. Quantum physicists talk about the energy of quanta, which is unseen energy, but it is full of potentials. I perceive complete health in the unseen quantum energy. We often do not realize complete health because we block it from our bodies. By being aware of it, feeling it, and keeping positive, we allow it to energize the potentials within our own cellular structures.

Another friend called shortly after this first healing I participated in and asked if I would pray and send healing energies for her nine-year-old nephew. He was seriously ill in a hospital and scheduled for surgery the next day. I lit a candle, became quiet, and focused for a time as I asked All That Is, the Source, to heal this little boy so he would not have to go through surgery. I felt then, and still do now in my work, very humble and sincere because of the trust others place in me to help pray for them. I again felt as if I were a conduit of energy when I asked for healing to come for this boy.

My friend and the boy's mother both called the next morning and told me that he did not have to have surgery after all, but the doctors could not explain why. This healing really awakened me to the fact that something must be happening. I was so naïve at the time. I did not know about energy, healing energies, therapeutic touch, or any of the other energy medicine modalities at that time. I think those phrases did not even exist. I knew of the healer Katherine Kuhlman from TV, and I remember very much wanting to be like her. The healings that came through her would bring tears to my eyes. Shortly after these two healing experiences of my own, I read the book *There Is a River,* by Thomas Sugrue, about the healings Edgar Cayce did, and that helped me to understand the healings that had just occurred.

After these two healing experiences, I knew that something must have happened through my intent and prayer and desire to be a conduit in healing. Science is just beginning to understand this sort of remote healing. (A good example of the power of prayer can be found in Larry Dossey's books on prayer and healing.) I decided, given my active, intuitive knowing and my experiences in helping others heal, that I would combine the two, and I dedicated my life to this work.

Some may say healing comes from being in a state of knowingness or simply in the Presence, which is where all healing exists. Though intuition seems to come naturally to me, I also nurture my intuitive abilities during my workday and stay tuned in to a healing flow. I take time between my sessions to enjoy a flow of well-being by listening to quiet meditative music, gazing at nature, or reflecting on how fortunate I am to be able to share these gifts with so many people who are in need of what I offer. When you appreciate what you have, you are given more, and I believe that is what keeps life moving, evolving.

Recently I worked with a young mother named Melinda. She told me of a myriad of physical disorders, all diagnosed by doctors. She had undergone numerous tests, from CT scans to blood tests. The doctors prescribed a list of medications, but the main diagnosis was stress. She asked me for help in reducing stress, as she did not want to take the prescription drugs. I suggested breathing techniques and visualizations to decrease her high stress levels, which she quickly accepted. Then she asked me to begin using healing energies in the remaining minutes of our first session.

As usual, when others ask for healing, I intuitively know what is going on with them. Melinda needed support for her immune system and her stressed adrenals. Her unmanaged stress had caused her cortisol levels to be extremely high, and she was moving toward a stroke or worse, as her stress was so out of control. We had a total of four sessions, and by the last, the frantic tremor in her voice had disappeared and she felt healed because some of the more severe issues had begun to fade away.

ENERGY PATTERNS AND NON-RESISTANCE

Sometimes my work consists of interpreting energy patterns in and around a client's energy fields so that I can determine what may be out of balance. Once that is done, I begin to energetically help correct the flow. For example, I worked with a client named George, who had developed severe headaches that happened only after he lay down to sleep. Neither physicians nor other health practitioners could give him a definitive answer as to the cause of the headaches.

Often a quantum field of energy is created during a conversation where healing is the serious intent of both parties. That intent was present George's case, and so we agreed to set an intention that he would surrender to healing energies. This non-resistance on a client's part helps me perceive what patterns need assistance in becoming healthy, vital energies. This is true whether they are mental, emotional, or physical energies.

Often, I find that a part of the body is ill or out of alignment because the person has been suffering inwardly for an indefinite period of time. As George surrendered, I was able to see what was creating the headaches. I was surprised at what I saw, which was some kind of brain injury—perhaps a sharp blow to his neck or some other incident in that general area—so I asked him about it. He confirmed that he had suffered a blow but had not connected that to the headaches, as nothing had ever shown up on tests. I saw that when he was in the prone position, there was not enough blood flow and oxygen to his head, and this seemed to cause his headaches.

Together we set the intention that more blood flow and oxygen could pass through his neck and into his brain. It is important for a client to agree and intend, as the body then follows the thought and begins to make new pathways and habits. I began to energetically focus on allowing for healing to take place; that is to say, I envisioned the narrowed parts of his spinal cord and arteries to the brain expanding so there would be more flow. George intended the same thing, and we both surrendered to the process.

Healing is really very simple: release resistance to well-being. We had three more sessions doing the same procedure, and George became free of the headaches that had plagued him.

Many people may find it unusual that these kinds of healings can take place at all, let alone over distances, but the facts speak for themselves. As you will read in the chapters that follow, my clients have experienced many different kinds of healings through the use of energy medicine.

5

Unconditional Desire and Healing a Wound

A hushed silence pervades the surroundings, and motion itself slows and becomes still. All things radiate forth an intense aliveness. Each is aware of every other. The luminous quality of the radiance is overwhelmingly Divine in nature.

—DAVID HAWKINS, *The Eye of the I*

Healers have played a role in society throughout recorded history. We find mention of spontaneous healing, healing that occurs without scientific explanation, in all religious traditions. Stories abound about healers who spend time talking with others and helping heal physical or emotional wounds, expand beliefs, and examine circumstances that could change for the better. By talking or praying with others with healing intent, and often by using the hands to direct energy, these healers act as focused channels for universal healing energy.

WHY SOME HEAL AND OTHERS DO NOT

Today many nurses, physicians, and other health professionals, like healers throughout the centuries, speak of a feeling that healing energy flows through them toward their patients. However, we often hear that the healer could not heal the patient. Why do some heal while others do not? It is simple, really. No one person can heal another. Healing is an interactive exchange of energy that must include an unconditional desire by the person who wants healing.

When there is illness, one must want to change something that led to it, and this has to occur before one can receive healing. There is nothing more powerful than one's own mind. The person desiring healing must be willing to let go of the past. Emotions and beliefs affect the physical body, as has been confirmed by science, especially quantum physics.

HEALTH PROFESSIONALS AND ENERGY MEDICINE

Today, healing that does not involve drugs, surgery, or other physical means is often called "energy medicine." This is the safest, most natural, and most accessible medicine, and it flows through all of us at all times. Shafica Karagulla, in *Breakthrough to Creativity,* writes about health professionals who intuitively know about dis-ease processes and who channel healing energy to their patients through intent and their hands, although their knowledge of higher-sensory perception is not something they often disclose to their colleagues, as they fear censure. I understand them from my own lifetime of intuitively seeing the blockages to health that cause illness in emotional and physical bodies. When those who desire healing ask me to help, I talk with them about their concerns and, when the time is right, begin the healing. Then I can feel the healing energy flow through me to the patient.

HEALING POTENTIAL AND ENERGY THREADS

Once the mind, emotions, and body have experienced a sense of health, either from engagement with a healer or through one's own efforts, and that person holds the potential of excellent health as his or her focus, realigning to health can be easy. This is so even if stress or negative thoughts begin to cause the mind and emotions, or even the body, to shift from balance to imbalance. Memory of a healthy experience acts to guide the way forward to health.

Most of those who have asked for my help desire healing at the deepest level and realize the importance of focus and commitment. Many create this desire after a conventional doctor gives an unfavorable medical prognosis and tells them that surgery, radiation, chemotherapy, or other drastic means are the only options. There are innumerable cases of those who have had healings through energy medicine after choosing it as their option.

During my first session with a new client, I may see any number of imbalances in the energy field that surrounds and moves through the body. As we agree to work together to bring balance, we talk not only about these imbalances, but also what the client has believed or experienced. Then, together we move the energy to clear up blockages, stuck memories, past stressful experiences, and even injuries.

One client, Shirley, called after she had an injury from taking a misstep and falling down a double flight of marble stairs. She sustained what at first appeared to be a blister on her shin, most likely from where it hit the edge of a stair, and her internist said there were no broken bones. However, two weeks later she was experiencing such discomfort that she went to an orthopedist for a second opinion. He found a fractured ankle, a torn ligament, and bone fragments as well as sepsis caused by an infection. Even with scrupulous care and strong antibiotics, a one-half-inch-deep wound was not healing.

Shirley went for three emergency room visits, and each time the diagnosis and recommendations, including hyperbaric and vacuum therapy, were scarier. The vacuum therapy would have required her to be attached to a suction device twenty-four hours a day for four to five weeks to draw out debris from the wound. With these prospects in front of her, Shirley listened as a friend, who was caring for her, told her about my column in the *Well Being Journal* and encouraged the woman to call me for help.

Shirley called me, and we agreed to work together over the phone. I began by energetically sensing her wound. With her permission, I started to see the tissue at the deepest part of her wound and then weave energetic threads across the area, in a manner similar to weaving strands of silk thread. The idea was to encourage the body's tissue to follow the path of the energetic weaving and repair itself. We worked together this way for five thirty-minute telephone sessions. She focused on the healing that she wanted to have, and I focused on energetically healing and stitching up the wound, from the deepest part to the surface.

At each of her checkups during this process, Shirley's doctors were surprised by how quickly this gaping wound in her leg was now healing. In fact, the doctor who had said she would need hyperbaric treatments reversed his stance. He said the wound was healing so nicely that she would not need the treatments after all, and she might not even need the plastic surgery he had originally predicted.

This is another case that substantiates the effectiveness of energy medicine. As more people experience energy medicine, they are discovering that it is not a new alternative, but rather a tried and true traditional medicine. One could say that energy medicine is a system of energies being applied to promote health, healing, and joy, and that energy is the medicine.

6

Self-Worth, Thoughts, Beliefs, and Stress

O, learn to read what silent love hath writ.

—SHAKESPEARE, ***Sonnet 23***

Intuition in medicine, in the healing and counseling professions, and in therapy in general is invaluable. The use of intuition helps the practitioner as well as the client to move forward beyond confusion, straight to the core of what stands in the way of healing. Intuitive insight helps me identify the essence of my clients' illnesses and then draw them out to talk about what I see occurring. During the course of the first conversation with almost all of my clients, I intuitively see an overview of the main issues they face that keep them from being healthier and happier.

Stress is the main factor in dis-ease causation. This fact is abundantly and unambiguously clear to me after working for more than forty-five years in the helping and healing professions. The largest contributors to stress are thoughts that do not feel good. You might ask, "Why would anyone think a thought that doesn't feel good?" No one deliberately thinks such thoughts. Rather, we do so habitually and subconsciously.

It may seem incongruous, but many people do not have enough self-worth to allow themselves to think thoughts that actually feel good. I have many clients who, during our conversations, demonstrate that they do not see themselves as being worthy of feeling good. I can sense when this is occurring.

For example, one of my clients, Karen, has a husband who always told her she was not being a good wife. Her difficulties worsened because she began to think of all the reasons why she was not good enough. She criticized herself about how she mothered her children, judged herself for not exercising enough, and blamed herself for not being calm enough. Her thoughts went directly to negative self-images just because her husband criticized her. It was my job to point this out to her, because she was not consciously focused on the fact that her thought processes were causing her discomfort and leading to more stress.

THINKING, BELIEVING, AND SELF-WORTH

As is true in the previous case, and in all others where thoughts are concerned, if you are thinking negative thoughts, you will need to monitor and stop them. Focus on thinking even the simplest thought that feels good. The reason for this is that negative thoughts change your body and brain chemistry immediately, raising tension and stress, which can create hormonal imbalances; positive, good-feeling thoughts decrease stress and create potential for greater health. Also, if you continue to think negative thoughts, a downward spiral of negativity can start attracting more such thoughts and beliefs. Biologist Bruce Lipton writes of the power of beliefs, which he discovered through his research: "Our perceptions, whether they are accurate or inaccurate, equally impact our behavior and our bodies. I celebrate the belief effect, which is an amazing testament to the healing ability of the body/mind."[1]

As I came to know Karen, my self-critical client, better, I intuitively saw her negative thought pattern regarding events she had scheduled, such as visits to her father. This woman had a history of critical abuse from her father and was afraid he would, as usual, openly criticize her in front of her children. She did not like to visit him because of this, but she knew he wanted to see his grandchildren. She would ultimately persuade herself to go because she felt she had to. She would regret it afterward, realizing that she could have chosen to do something else, such as focus on other priorities that would bring her joy.

MAKE SIMPLE CHANGES FIRST

Karen realized she had to do something. The change she needed to make was very simple, but I wondered if she would do it. When you think even the simplest, most general positive thought, such as, "I'm happy the sun is shining today," you begin an upward spiral of positive thoughts; then, thinking more such thoughts becomes easier. Like attracts like.

Start simply, because you do not want to say "I'm such a wonderful person" when you are feeling self-critical or do not really believe you are wonderful at the moment. Instead, find one small thing to focus on, such as, "I just prepared a wonderful meal for my family." Then you are focused on a positive thing about yourself.

Karen wanted to feel better about herself, but she was unsure how to do it. When we first started working together, she was nervous and would laugh at the end of every sentence. I noticed this, of course, and discovered what was behind it all. When she was young, Karen was met with constant criticism. Her father was extremely critical, and she took in his harsh words, which led her to lose her self-confidence. Her father was an alcoholic, cruel and insulting, and at an early age she developed the thought habit of holding many negative images of herself.

As an adult, every time Karen visited her father, she feared his criticism. I used a lot of different tools with her, including visualizing safe zones, in order to help build her self-esteem step by step. One of my initial suggestions was for her to keep in mind that when someone criticizes her or complains about her, it is really all about that person being in a negative state. When someone attacks you, verbally or otherwise, it is really about their issues, and how you respond to them is up to you. The bottom line is that it is imperative that everyone generates self-worth. Self-worth can come from a sense of compassion toward, for example, people who are out of sorts and casting blame on those around them. You can reason, "If so-and-so is blaming me, he (or she) must be having a difficult time."

Children are naturally happy and healthy. But from childhood, when we are frisky and happy and do not really care what others think, we inherit beliefs from our culture, our tribe, and our family that limit us. Some of these exhortations may sound familiar: "What would people think?" "Don't be so selfish." "Don't share your things with others." "There is not enough to go around." "Don't talk back." "No one will ever like you if you are like that." "Only speak when spoken to."

Karen held many of these beliefs, but perhaps judged herself more harshly than many others would judge themselves. With my encouragement, she started to write a list of her good qualities and began to realize these were real once she focused on writing them. She perceived that she is a good person, a good mother, a good wife, and an intelligent individual. We worked together on having her really feel the truth of these qualities; we had to do this on a very deep level in order for her to change her beliefs. She started understanding that she needed to feel more compassion for her father; she gradually started taking his behavior less personally and started seeing him in a better light.

We also worked on how these changes in Karen affected her relationship with her husband. When someone who has not had positive self-esteem starts to gain it, those in relationship with this person will sense the change and want to make adjustments as well. Things have improved in Karen's marriage, and her husband has adjusted to her more positive nature.

Self-worth means you take care of yourself and do not allow others to walk all over you. Recently another client, Helen, told me her husband suggested they get divorced because she was not a good housekeeper and she was not taking care of herself. She grew up with parental criticism, similar to Karen's situation. She took on this criticism and then had thoughts and feelings of unworthiness throughout her life. It was as though these thoughts magnetically attracted criticism from Helen's husband. She does not have to work or think about any career because her husband provides a nice income, and she felt it imperative that she build up her feelings of self-worth in order to create a successful marriage.

BELIEF FORMATION AND PERPETUATION

Helen's lack of self-worth seemed to be all she knew about herself. It is important to know that a belief is formed simply from a particular thought a person keeps thinking. Helen kept reinforcing her beliefs by embracing the criticisms from her parents and husband that she was not good enough to be happy, to take it easy, to have the things she wanted. She, like Karen, especially dreaded visiting her continually critical parents with her husband and children.

Helen had a belief that she must regularly do something or be some way that did not ultimately feel good to her. I worked with Helen to help her change her beliefs and to see how they had developed over time. I helped her realize that by choosing positive thoughts, she could turn negative beliefs into positive ones. You really rule your own life this way from both your physical and spiritual nature.

Gradually she came to realize that she—and everyone else—is completely worthy to feel good every minute of life. Self-respect is the outcome of choosing thoughts that feel good or are fun to think. Practicing the thought "I am completely worthy" can help you embrace the feeling of self-worth, but you have to believe it in order for the thought to have an effect on your body.

Why was it so easy for my clients to feel unworthy? It was easy because for most of their lives they had practiced the thought—whether subtly or consciously—of being unworthy, as many of us have done from childhood. When I was a child, I accepted the belief that I was unworthy, whether it stemmed from a dogma or a comment from a parent or other adult. I had to realize, as Helen did, that I had to change my beliefs with regard to basic worthiness.

We are all worthy simply by being alive. However, we have to stop limiting ourselves by the thoughts we think. When we believe limited things about ourselves, such as that we are unworthy to be happy or take it easy or be successful, it is as if we agree with the limits. We thus attach ourselves to limited identities by our thoughts and beliefs and do not feel free to grow.

Helen realized she had dug a hole for herself in this regard. She was depressed and knew things were spiraling downward. I intuitively knew she was reacting to her husband, and men in general, in the same way she reacted to her parents. When I told her that I saw this happening, she responded well and wanted to know what to do to change her reactions. I told her, as I had Karen, that if she started changing her thoughts and beliefs, she would feel better about herself. As a result, she would more likely be able to visit her parents and not let their negative comments pull her down into despair. We worked on building her self-esteem by having her create a strong desire to start feeling better about herself. To my delight, she did so and made improvements, which I intuitively knew she could do, just as I had.

SELF-RESPECT, FORGIVENESS, AND ALIGNMENT

I suggested to Helen that she make a list of the critical things she remembered her parents saying and then practice forgiving herself for believing them, as forgiveness is a way to align to the powerful feeling of absolute self-worth. I had also asked Karen to focus on seeing that she was worthy of being appreciated, despite her father's words. Both clients made their lists, did their self-forgiveness, and then started the work of appreciating themselves for the loving and unique individuals they are. Helen also made other changes. She and her husband are much happier, and she also has continued, independently, to do her own personal work.

RESPECT, THOUGHTS, AND FEELINGS

Our bodies want to be happy and serve us. What is it that so often gets in the way of the body actually being healthy and happy in a consistent way? It is partly because of our negative thoughts and emotions that we are led to feel lack of self-worth. By not listening to our bodies and our feelings and monitoring our thoughts, we turn away from being happy. What thoughts and emotions prevent the flow of well-being for our bodies? Are we doing something that we do not like in order to meet someone else's approval? That cannot feel good, and what does not feel good becomes a challenge for the body. Self-respect is central to being healthy. When you respect your body and the spark within you—your spirit—life becomes much easier.

It is important to remember that we inherit a lot of negativity from the time we are born, as relatives and many others attempt to mold us into their reality. Limiting rules, rules that make sense in some contexts but not others, and even self-imposed limits, often keep us from feeling the joy of life flowing through us at all times. When that flow is limited, then illnesses can begin to manifest; the body likes us to be happy, and when we are not, immunity is compromised to the extent that our good feelings are not allowed to flow.

7

A Case Demonstrating the Reversal of Cellular Stress

The Importance of Positive Thought and Emotion

Your time is limited, so don't waste it living someone else's life. . . . Don't be trapped by dogma, which is living with the results of other people's thinking. Don't let the noise of others' opinions drown out your own inner voice. Most important, have the courage to follow your heart and intuition. They somehow already know what you truly want to become. Everything else is secondary.

—STEVE JOBS, *Time Magazine*

Stress. The word has myriad negative connotations. It has accumulated numerous meanings over the past thirty-plus years, being used to describe everything from enormous anxiety to extreme physical overload. It is unresolved stress, however, that causes problems, as it can lead to cardiovascular and other major dis-eases, insomnia, adrenal dysfunction, blood sugar imbalances including diabetes, and, at times, complete inability to function in even the smallest of daily activities.

STRESS AND THOUGHT CHOICES

Our greatest resource for resolving stress is our power to choose the thoughts we think. Our thoughts affect our bodies from their minutest molecules to all their larger systems. Thoughts often precede emotions, and research has proven, beyond any reasonable doubt, that human emotions have a direct influence on the way our cells behave and function. The work of biologist Candace Pert provides well-known substantiation for the fact that emotions guide molecules, and her book *Molecules of Emotion* is worth reading. We also know, from the work of geneticists and their research (some of which is described in Dawson Church's excellent book *The Genie in Your Genes*), that our DNA can be shifted and changed by our thoughts. As thoughts affect emotions, both of which are immediately read by the minutest parts of the body, we do well to think the best of ourselves and others.

For example, we know that negative thoughts and emotions can do such things as raise cortisol levels; cortisol is the stress hormone made by the adrenal glands. Chronic negative or stressful thinking ultimately will adversely affect the function of the adrenal glands themselves. To be sure, there is a positive kind of stress, where anyone can use stimuli in the environment as a challenge. This can take the form of channeling one's energy to complete a project or do something that seems difficult but would bring a positive outcome once done. The completion of a task creates an inertia that helps one continue on in a creative mode. It also raises levels of endorphin, the feel-good molecule; athletes often experience this increase in endorphins during workouts and competitions.

Athletes use a kind of positive stress that may seem very challenging at the time of greatest focus, but that ultimately leads to a very positive feeling of completion. As another example, imagine getting to an airport and going through screening in time to catch a particular flight. This could be seen as a negative stress, but the anticipation and satisfaction of being in your airplane seat, soon to arrive at your chosen destination, could be seen as a positive stress.

It is a situation that is well worth "jumping through the hoops." We can focus on positive outcome in the midst of stress.

Students have more dental issues around exam times, and I remember how my own gums bled when I was in graduate school, all due to cramming at the last minute and worrying. I learned that if I had been more diligent in my ongoing studies, I would not have experienced such last-minute stress. Consistently taking adequate vitamins and minerals, amino acids, and other nutrients our bodies require while staying away from junk food could help us in those times of stress, as our bodies can bounce back more rapidly to states of health and harmony.

The stress experienced by those who have lost their jobs or their homes can be similar to those who have experienced loss due to floods, tornadoes, and hurricanes. None of these stressors are in the preferred reality, but on some level they must be accepted so that we can somehow move forward in our lives. People everywhere on our planet are finding themselves in extraordinarily stressful situations. It seems that only a minority of people have found personal tools to move forward independently into more peaceful circumstances without the loving assistance of others; fortunately, there are many dedicated helpers who give of themselves to help others in their times of need, as we have all witnessed during the aftermath of natural and man-made disasters.

CHRONIC NEGATIVE STRESS, EMOTIONS, AND THE BODY

Chronic emotional stress is a different story. This is the kind of stress that is unresolved, so even if it is subconscious, it continues to cause physical stress and even resistance to the natural healing rhythms for the cells of the body. Following is a case study illustrating how stress affects the cells in the body. First, however, I refer to biophysicist Joyce Whiteley Hawkes, who writes beautifully of the intelligence of the cells. She writes,

> Cells are the foundation of physical life. Groups of cells form tissues, and similar tissues join together and form organs, which are dependent on the health of underlying cells.
>
> Individually, cells are small: ten thousand can fit on the head of a pin. . . . Within each cell there are trillions of molecules composed of trillions more atoms. Like the spaces between stars, which contain huge amounts of energy, the ultrasmall nano-spaces inside of the atoms team with energy to constantly manifest new creation. In this microworld of the inner composition of your cells, energy and matter interface in ultrafast blips of time: nano- or pico-seconds. When an event occurs in these swift pulses of 10^{-9} or 10^{-12} seconds, the cells enter a type of quantum reality—no longer linear and no longer predictable. The cell is the interface between ordinary and nonordinary reality; possibilities exist here that we have barely begun to understand or develop. . . . Yet we can influence them with our consciousness. [1]

Hawkes' description of cells not only helps our understanding of them, but also highlights the importance of visualizing their ability to remain in the flow of health. Our thoughts, our consciousness, is not disconnected from our cells. Each thought and emotion instantaneously affects all of our trillions upon trillions of cells and everything in them, from mitochondria to DNA. Chronically held negative thoughts and emotions have the deepest effect on our health; researchers such as Hans Selye think the chronic stress from these unseen energies causes almost 100 percent of dis-ease.

Following is a case that describes the cells of the body from my perspective in intuitive medicine and illustrates how cells react to chronic, unmanaged stress. I mention the adrenal glands first because, most often, they are the first of the body's systems to be affected by chronic stress. The cardiovascular system follows, then the thyroid, which often is hypoactive if stress has long been unmanaged. Next is the esophagus, which is often affected by gastroesophageal reflux dis-ease (GERD).

What I see and do can be illustrated by Wanda's case. She called because, as she said, "I feel like my entire body is inflamed," She added, "I've been under enormous stress for the last twelve months." She described the situation, but I felt there was something she was not saying that was affecting her deeply. I also discovered that Wanda was being denied access to her grandchildren due to a family conflict, and this caused her great, ongoing stress.

I could immediately see how Wanda's unresolved stress, her continual thinking of stressful thoughts, had weakened the adrenals and led to GERD. As I talked her, I began energetically working. I immediately started the virtual healing process on the affected areas (with permission, of course). How this physical manifestation of emotional stress showed up in Wanda's adrenal cells and glands is the same process as in all cases of chronic stress.

I always see clumps of trillions of dark cells in stressed areas of the body; the cells are dark because of the stress. When you think of the description of the cells given by Hawkes, you can imagine how all the parts she describes—the molecules and atoms, the space in between them, as well as the mitochondria, the chromosomes, the DNA, and more—take on the effects of thought and emotion. I see how they begin to shut down when our thoughts and emotions are cut off from the ease of well-being, from thinking thoughts of wellness or happiness. The systems renew and are vital, as if guided by some extremely intelligent source, when we do not block the flow of health by negative, stressful thinking and related emotions.

In Wanda's case, the constant difficult emotions she held from the thoughts of her family situation and her feelings of distress, resentment, and fear had caused the cells to start to dysfunction. When trillions upon trillions of the cells begin to dysfunction and this occurs day after day because of unresolved or chronic stress, then the distress begins to manifest. The adversely affected cells become numerous enough that they begin to form clumps and start to block the natural processes of the glands and other systems. These dark cells I see in my clients were previously healthy cells that had been full of light and in healthy function. The mitochondria, the DNA and genetic structure, and the messenger molecules were all working healthfully. When there is stress, this entire cellular system is blocked from the natural flow of health and begins to shut down. The cells begin to proliferate in their dysfunctional state if the consistent negative thoughts and emotions continue over a period of time.

It is important to focus on the desired outcome of not only helping someone change his or her thoughts and emotions toward those of wellness, appreciation, and abundance, but also helping the body to generate trillions of new, healthy cells. The body responds immediately, as soon as the thoughts and emotions change. The body cannot hold a thought frequency of illness when the person holds thoughts that have a higher frequency of love and appreciation. It is a matter of focus; you cannot focus on someone you love and feel hate at the same time. I have long worked with clients to facilitate their bodies in building trillions upon trillions of new, healthy cells in this way as well as through focusing healing energies to assist the process.

For example, it was clear that Wanda's adrenals needed immediate support, and I began a process of entering in consciousness into her adrenals and supporting, through healing intent, thought, and imagery, the building of new cells based on the original healthy blueprint of her DNA. Sometimes the way I do this is to imagine I am using a brush-like instrument that paints on trillions of healthy cells, all based on the original, healthy, genetic blueprint of the client.

Our thoughts do affect our DNA. It is as if our DNA is listening to each thought and emotion for instructions on whether to replicate healthy cells or compromised cells. As I work with the client's body to encourage it to build trillions of healthy cells, at the same time I am helping the body wash away the dark cells that had responded to the thoughts and emotions of chronic stress. But my primary focus is on helping the body to generate and accept the new, healthy, bright, life-filled cells. As part of this process, the telomeres—the end points of the genes—which determine cellular health and longevity in the remaining healthy cells, also become more energized. Along with all that, I find that making sure my clients understand the vital role they play in supporting their DNA with thoughts of wellness is of central importance.

THE POWER OF SELF-FORGIVENESS

When I have second and third sessions with clients, I can sometimes see that the original work, which began to help the body build new, healthy cells, has not held up. At this point I ask them what has been occurring in their lives since the most recent session, and there are always some negative thoughts or emotional patterns that have recurred. This, in turn, curtails the work we had done in the previous session. So again I help them go through the process of letting go of these thoughts and feelings; this takes more practice if one has not done so, and most often it involves self-forgiveness. Usually, when I see the work is not progressing quite so well, I ask my clients how they are doing with self-forgiveness.

For example, I talked with a client who was more energized than she had been in the previous session; she seemed to have made a shift toward more positive thinking. She reported that the more she had practiced self-forgiveness, the easier it had become to align with good-feeling thoughts. Her recovery had progressed because she had corrected her negative thinking. The principle of self-forgiveness is mainly to forgive yourself for judgments you have placed on yourself; as you recall your negative thoughts and feelings about yourself, you take a moment and, really feeling it, say something like, "Despite the fact that I have thought this about myself, I now let go of it and deeply love and completely accept myself." And you do the same for those judgments or criticisms you have placed on others and on circumstances and events, whether recent or from as far back as you can remember. Forgiveness can be said to be the same as aligning with healthy thinking about a past situation or thinking of what you want that will feel better.

Forgiveness releases negative energies and allows the natural flow of well-being to bathe your cells and, therefore, your entire body. It is perhaps one of the most important processes you can do for your own health on an ongoing basis—at least until you have mastered thought and think well of yourself and others 100 percent of the time.

8

Old Beliefs, Emotions, and Intuitional Perception for Healing

One's thoughts, especially when amplified by intent or emotion, leave an imprint on matter; that is, will directs all energy.

—VALERIE HUNT, *Infinite Mind*

My clients sometimes ask me about the process by which I intuitively receive information from them when they ask me to help them heal. I have a broad understanding of anatomy from my work in hospice and other professions as well as more than forty years of medical intuitive and healing work. This knowledge helps me immeasurably in receiving visual images from the physical bodies of my clients. I also perceive similar information from the emotional field. A strong belief or habit of thought is easy to see in the field, and such patterns play a significant role in overall health.

HOLDING ONTO MEMORIES AND PHYSICAL DIS-EASE

A client named John called me several weeks after undergoing back surgery, from which he had somewhat recovered. During my initial scanning of his body and his emotional field, I sensed clearly that he was holding onto some very difficult memories and emotions from events that had taken place years before, when he was in high school. I sensed he was ready to let go of these old thoughts. I could feel his heartache, which stemmed from his belief that he was unworthy to be a normal, whole person, although he had a strong desire to be such a person.

As I focused, I also received the impression that he had allowed himself to be injured—and that this had to do with his feeling that he was not whole and worthy just as he was. I could hear in his voice and see from the cloudy images in his emotional field (indicative of self-sabotage) that he was looking for attention from his mother. He confirmed all of this verbally as our session continued.

John started courting injuries when he was young and continued as he went through medical school, then law school, and even as he began practicing law. His low self-esteem contributed to poor physical and emotional health and lack of success in his profession. Later he told me that when he was ill or injured, his mother would rush—via train or airplane, if necessary—to his side, no matter where in the world he was. He had used physical injuries in several ways to get attention from his mother, who had always been very busy with her own life—except when her son had a medical emergency of some kind.

I was struck by the intensity of his willingness to be injured or ill in order to receive special attention from someone. He was not the first person with this syndrome whom I had counseled, but he was certainly the most open and honest; he took responsibility for wanting and needing what I would call normal attention, and he acknowledged having resorted to some drastic steps in order to get it. John had not had an emotionally healthy relationship with either of his parents, and early on he had learned to find his emotional comfort through injuries. He even found pleasure in the attention he received from nurses, doctors, and aides when he was in the emergency room or surgical unit.

I could see where his injuries and surgeries had taken quite a toll on his body and spirit. I told him the first step in climbing out of the hole of neediness and becoming full and complete within his own self was to forgive himself. We are taught to forgive others, but the truth is that we can never truly do so until we forgive ourselves. We must first forgive ourselves for judging, feeling neglected, being resentful of others, and holding negative emotions in any circumstance in order for forgiveness to open us to feeling worthy and allowing the flow of well-being that is always available from Source.

John did the forgiveness work for himself and realized immediate emotional healing. Then, during our last session, he asked for healing for his left leg, which he said felt numb, very weak, and slightly cold compared to his other leg.

KNITTING DAMAGED PARTS BACK TOGETHER AGAIN

Here is another explanation of how healing work can be done. As I focus on body parts or systems such as the nerves, I receive very definite impressions. It is as if I am looking through a high-powered, lighted microscope when I focus on the area that needs help; where there is a need to knit together damaged nerves, veins, arteries, bones, or skin, I perceive a brightly lit area at a microscopic level. Even though nerves are tiny, they look very large to me as I knit parts back together. I see the cells coming together, and I energetically encourage healthy cells into place with my client's cooperation. The combination of intents—the client's and mine—is what allows healing so quickly.

After I had worked for a while in this way, John, sounding surprised, said that his upper leg and knee felt noticeably warmer. I kept the healing energies flowing, and he soon laughed and said, "My toes are warm again!" I then asked him if there was any reason for his leg to return to being cold (such as his need for attention), and he emphatically said "No!" but added that he would call me again if he needed any help. However, I doubt that he will, as I think he reached a milestone by forgiving himself and realizing he did not need anyone's attention in order to feel good about himself.

Another example of the clear impressions I get from scanning my clients' physical and emotional fields can be seen in Ellen's case. During our first healing session, which was over the phone, I scanned Ellen's body at her request. As I do with most clients, I started at her head and worked downward; working in this way, I perceive various injuries—many from early childhood, others from later accidents or physical abuse.

I see visual impressions as I scan; for example, I can see if there has been a fracture because a line where the fracture occurred comes into my visual field as I scan that location. As I continue to scan, I assess the various glands, organs, bones, joints, and discs throughout the body, and often one or more of them will start flashing. What this means is that I get a visual impression if there is something out of order, whether from the past, the present, or likely to occur soon. During the scan, I also tend to see how a person's emotions influence his or her body.

I was scanning Ellen's body and reporting to her what I saw when she interrupted me to say that she had had an appointment earlier in the week with her doctor, who had given her several diagnoses. She said that I was seeing and confirming everything he had said. It makes me feel wonderful when I get feedback like this, because then I know I am still perceiving these things accurately.

9

The Importance of Letting Go of Unwanted Conditions

> ***On an emotional level, healing means releasing what tethers us to our sense of separateness, of being wronged, superior, inferior, lacking, and so on. It means giving up our habits of resistance and "against-ness," whether they are being directed toward our spouses, our bosses, our children, our parents, our friends, the government, corporations, or most especially, toward life.***
>
> **—Leigh Fortson, *Embrace, Release, Heal***

One of the most important issues in healing is embodied in this question: "Are you ready to let go of your issues?" or, put another way, "Are you ready for a complete healing of any and all illnesses?" I ask all my clients to consider this question in the healing work we do together. The more a person is committed to his or her own healing, the more effective the one who helps the person heal can be.

I can intuitively feel the shift when a client lets go of his or her issues; it is as if the energy of the illness dissolves. Each client is unique; however, when he or she is focused on healing, unconditional love plays a big role in establishing a relationship of trust, not only with the healer, but also with life itself. That trust is the bedrock of the letting go of illness, after which healing begins. At this point, it is important that the client stay focused on the healing rather than on any physical or emotional condition.

CONDITIONS CHANGE WITH LETTING GO

The condition will change with the letting go and the focus on the healing, and I look for each client's desire to participate in these. I once worked with Brenda, who was having pain with every step she took due to a growth between her big toe and the next toe. I intuitively saw little tentacles spreading out and grabbing onto nerves and bones in her foot. She could see and feel the hard bump at the center, and it was very painful to the touch. It met the descriptions of a ganglion or a neuroma.

I asked Brenda if she was ready to let go and to heal, and she indicated she was. I then asked her to place her first and second fingers on the bump ever so lightly and to focus on healing. I also focused on her healing by energetically placing my fingers over hers.

In just a few minutes she exclaimed, "I can feel the bump getting softer already!" and we continued. A few minutes later, Brenda said that the bump was almost gone, and a short time after that she said, "The bump is gone! I can't feel anything abnormal there at all."

Often the healing process can seem like a miracle or, as it is sometimes called in medicine, a spontaneous remission, but it is really just a matter of alignment and energy focus, and letting go of previous conditions.

I asked Brenda to take a few steps, and when she did, she said the pain was gone, the bump was gone, and her foot felt normal again. We spoke about how important it was for her to continue to let go of negative thoughts and attitudes and to focus on the bright side of life. This successful case of healing speaks once again about how personal participation makes all the difference and how truly important it is to have a "clean slate."

10

The Healing Power of Forgiveness

Like love, joy is fearless and untroubled by the world. . . . Joy does not come and go; what comes and goes is our awareness of joy.

—ROBERT HOLDEN, *Be Happy*

A client named Kathy told me of an experience that illustrates how powerful forgiveness can be for healing a physical condition. Kathy lives in the same town I do, and she was very aware of my therapy practice and the importance I place on doing forgiveness work for oneself. As I often explain, we cannot forgive anyone or anything outside of ourselves until we first forgive ourselves for judgments and negative emotions. It is often a very challenging process, perhaps one of the most difficult we have to do. Only after forgiving ourselves, and then others, can true healing take place.

I know Kathy to be a very balanced person who rarely judges anyone or anything. She has had a lifetime of doing forgiveness work, and she has done it impeccably. Recently she purchased a new car, which her husband, Sean, had agreed would be for her. She would make the payments, and Sean was happy with the arrangement.

In one of our sessions, Kathy related that one night Sean had suggested they eat out, as they had both worked hard all day and neither of them wanted to prepare a meal. Kathy agreed and said she would drive; however, Sean insisted that he drive. She thought to herself, "Well, it won't hurt to let him drive this time," and she gave in. Sean drove while she thought of a nice place to unwind from the week.

Suddenly she realized Sean was driving to a place where she was not comfortable eating, as the previous three times she ate there, she had suffered from varying degrees of food poisoning. She said, "I don't want to eat there. Don't you remember? Let's go somewhere else." Sean insisted, however, saying, "But it's inexpensive." Kathy protested again, but by that time Sean had parked the car and turned off the engine. She thought, "He doesn't care what I think, and he doesn't care about my stomach!"

BEING IN TOUCH WITH YOUR FEELINGS

I asked Kathy what her feelings had been at that time. She said she had been unhappy that she was at a place she preferred not to be, and she was there because Sean had not cared about the type of food she ate. She said she had been frustrated with Sean's insensitivity to her.

Parked at the restaurant, Kathy exited the passenger side of her new car. Just as she pushed the door shut, her wristwatch became caught on a projection on the door jamb. The door slammed on her left hand, which was caught horizontally between the door and the jamb. The force of the door closing broke her thumb, smashed her knuckles together, and broke her wrist. Her hand was crushed from her little finger across the knuckles to her thumb, and her wrist was twisted by her watch, still caught on the door.

Kathy told me that, in hindsight, she realized she could have asked Sean to stop the car that night in order to make a decision agreeable to both of them about where to eat. She thought over the event again, saying she had unhooked the seatbelt and stepped out of the car, and her wristwatch caught on the car as she shut the door. I sensed there was more emotion involved in the incident and asked her about that. She said she wondered if she had subconsciously pushed the door shut a little harder than normal; she also wondered why her wristwatch had caught on the car just as the door was being shut.

Because she was in shock and pain, she had not been thinking rationally at that time. She had thought to herself, "I can get through this," and began to walk to the restaurant behind her husband. She had blocked the pain and acted as if nothing had taken place, although her left hand and wrist looked disfigured. She told me that her mind-over-matter efforts had worked for a time. She had reasoned that many people have been healed with this very attitude, so why not her?

Ultimately, Sean took her to the ER at the local hospital late that evening as she dealt with the severe pain of a fractured thumb and wrist. Once several X-rays had been taken and her arm, fingers, and thumb had been stabilized with a splint, they went home. Kathy was in excruciating pain for days, and pain medications could not help much, since they made her nauseated.

RELIVING UNPLEASANT MEMORIES AND FORGIVING

When I called Kathy for her next appointment, she said she had begun to replay the events of that evening two or three days into her pain- and house-ridden state, and what she had started to understand was not peaceful for her. I asked her if she had forgiven herself and her husband. She said she had started the process but knew there was more forgiveness work to do.

Kathy's review of her visit to the ER was a crucial piece in this story, as it was there that she realized she had forgiveness work to do. She said the X-ray technician at the ER had marveled at the odd shape of her wrist and thumb and the position of her hand. The pain was severe, and he radiology report showed fractures. When a clinician placed Kathy's hand and wrist in a splint and wrapped it in an Ace bandage in preparation for a visit to an orthopedic doctor a few days later, she thought about starting serious forgiveness work as soon as she could.

Kathy said she knew she had to begin by forgiving herself for allowing a self-inflicted injury to happen, even though it had been unintended. She said, "It was just one of those things that happen." I believe that. Sometimes these things just happen, and we learn from them. Once she knew she had forgiven herself for allowing the injury, she realized she then had to forgive herself for not asserting herself more directly that evening with Sean. When done with that, Kathy knew she had to forgive her husband for not listening to her, for not being sensitive to her food preferences, and for taking her to a restaurant he knew she did not like. She noted that she did her work assiduously, knowing she had to so that the experience would not begin affecting her in a negative manner.

Four days after our session, Kathy visited the orthopedic doctor's office, and her wrist, hand, and thumb were subsequently placed in a brace she had to wear for six to eight weeks. At our next session, she said that her pain was still severe. I sensed even more work was necessary, and Kathy confirmed this by saying she had a deep feeling that more profound work at a deeper level would help healing in all areas of her life. She began to focus more and more on self-forgiveness and, with an intense desire, set the intention to stay with the process until she felt totally free of any judgment and negative thoughts or feelings regarding her husband, herself, and anyone else whom she might have judged.

At her next doctor visit a week later, the orthopedist took more X-rays. Shortly thereafter, he walked into the room where she waited and, with a smile and a puzzled look on his face, said that he did not see any fractures of her wrist or thumb. He told her to wiggle her fingers, continue wearing the brace, and come back in three more weeks.

I saw the X-rays—the before and after—and can testify that it was true: within one week's time, the fractures were healed. Her doctor's explanation for this anomaly was that it might have just been arthritis. Yet he had before him two X-rays taken a week apart, with the first showing fractures and the second showing none.

SURRENDER AND HEALING

Kathy and I discussed what might have led to this amazing healing of fractures in one week. She said she thought it was not only the forgiveness work she had done so profoundly, but also the fact that she had surrendered. As she rested at home, she simply surrendered to her present condition while allowing the state of healing that came with the forgiveness work. This is so true; it is when you allow the healing forces of nature to act, when you are in the state of presence that forgiveness offers, that natural healing takes place so well. It is only unusual to heal so dramatically because of our belief that it is not normal.

In my experience of working with people on a deep level, I have found that a sincere dedication to "doing the work" must take place for healing to really settle in. Many times people say they do not know where to begin, and I always say, "Start at the beginning. Simply say to yourself, 'I forgive myself,' and repeat it until a thought or image comes to mind. Work with that one until you feel clear, and then silently forgive the outer circumstance or person related to that image." This helps you align to positive thought, which is healing.

It is very important to keep on keeping on, especially if you have a deep torment of the soul or are suffering physically from an illness that was created from a negative mental or emotional state or experience. Tears may flow, and they can be welcomed as a cleansing of the emotions. Anger can be released through tears as well as through the visualization of an event so that the healing of anger can happen through forgiveness. ("I forgive myself for being in fear" is one example of what you might say during forgiveness practice. You might also say, "Despite the fact that I had fear, I forgive myself now and deeply love and completely accept myself." This leads to a deep love and acceptance of others along with forgiveness and realignment with positive thinking).

Our bodies reflect our thoughts and feelings, and we can trace illnesses to negativity of some kind. Self-forgiveness can be a short path to peace if it is done with sincerity and a pure heart. And, as Kathy's experience shows, forgiveness leads to powerful healing of body and mind.

11

Anxiety, Depression, and the Power of Talk Therapy with Energy Medicine

What matters to you? Are your thoughts aligned with what matters to you? Are your behaviors aligned with what matters to you?

—Eric Maisel, Rethinking Depression

Even the worst cases of depression and anxiety are responsive to treatment. Energy medicine and talk therapy can be the most powerful aids, but certainly nutritional changes can help, as well. Many people are deficient in oxytocin, a neurotransmitter released in the brain during positive social connections and loving touch. Everyone needs encouragement, a hug, positive input, a nice pat on the back, or even a big smile, any of which can change one's outlook on life. There is evidence that newborn babies, especially premature babies in neonatal units, need to be held or they can develop a condition called "failure to thrive." This is also true of patients of all ages in skilled nursing facilities and hospitals. There is no place with more depressed people than a facility where there are no visitors or others to communicate some form of positive feedback each day.

LACK OF NURTURING

Oxytocin levels rise in the body from touch therapies, including non-contact therapeutic touch (NCTT) and energy medicine. This neurotransmitter has been found to be very low in those who are depressed. Lack of nurturing touch can be a central cause of anxiety and depression. Many people may not even recognize that they are anxious or depressed and often blame their symptoms or feelings on something entirely different from the actual cause.

Interestingly, I see anxiety and depression in many of my clients before they have identified it themselves. They may call me for other reasons, but during our appointments, I intuitively sense many things in their lives. I use the phrase "energy medicine" to encompass my work not only using medical intuition, but also directing healing energies, something we can all do by focusing the will.

The effectiveness of energy medicine is based on the fact that we are all energetically connected in a quantum energy field. This is why I, as well as others, can assist with healing at a distance. I do ninety percent of my work by telephone, and thousands of my clients have had healings. Here is a statement from one of my clients attesting to this power of connection that transcends what is seen:

> I noticed an unusual mole appear on my arm. It grew very rapidly, reaching a quarter-inch in diameter. I called Shannon McRae because I had heard of her healing work, and I told her about the mole. She said, "Okay, will you put your finger on the spot?" I did. Then she said, "Now I am going to put my finger energetically over yours. Can you feel that?" And I did! I said, "Yes, I feel it," as I could feel a warm tingling. Then she said, "Okay, now the energy that created the growth is gone. Can you feel that?"
>
> I felt a tingling sensation and a release of a very subtle energy, and, of course, I wanted it to be gone, too, so I'm sure I played a role. I was thinking that "wherever two or more are gathered in spirit" for a purpose, our spirit would assist, and I truly believed it! Within days, I noticed the mole begin to decrease in size, and in a little more than a month, it was gone! It has now been a year and there is no sign of anything but smooth skin.

This case, which I will describe in more detail in the next chapter, demonstrates an outcome that I have seen time and again for more than forty years. Energy medicine works. Much scientific evidence validates the effectiveness of healing energy. Recently, for example, researchers at the Rhine Research Center found that healers who channel energy show evidence of producing energy at a far higher rate than normal. Using a multiphasic ultraviolet light detector designed to measure individual photons produced per half-second, the researchers measured dramatic increases in the number of photons in a room when healers performed healing sessions. Another study showed that those treated with NCTT demonstrated a greater decrease in anxiety than those who had no contact with a healer or other helper.[1]

THE BODY DOES NOT KNOW THE DIFFERENCE BETWEEN IMAGINATION AND REALITY

Repetitive negative thinking and physical illness may be the most common causes of depression and the most important to first examine. Many people do not realize that the thoughts they think cause their bodies to have immediate emotional reactions. A simple habit of thought, such as reliving an uncomfortable memory, anticipating a negative outcome, or obsessing about a relationship challenge, can cause depression. The body does not know the difference between imagining negative things and the reality of them; it reacts to both the same way. Gloomy emotions can begin to take over with chronic negative thinking. This is when many people start to become increasingly unhappy, forlorn, or sad. Then, with time or repeated negative thinking, they become mildly, moderately, or severely depressed. In fact, I sense some depression in almost everyone who calls.

Another cause of depression can be concern about a physical illness. Often a person may have just a nebulous feeling about an illness that is unbalancing his or her life, but I can sense depression in people like this, even if they cannot quite define it themselves. In these cases, as with all my clients, I begin by being open with them and asking how I can help.

SIGNS OF DEPRESSION

Signs of depression can include constant despondency or sadness, continual tiredness, insomnia, inability to get to sleep easily, excessive time spent sleeping, weight gain, overeating or poor appetite, difficult or uninspiring relationships, a feeling that life is not worthwhile or is too much of a struggle, feelings of hopelessness or unworthiness, an inability to move forward, agitation, and a sense that everything is falling apart.

Depression can also be caused by circumstances such as the loss of a friend, relative, pet, or job; ill health; recent diagnosis of an illness; and chronic pain. Always, the attitude a person has about everything plays a key role. While thought is the most important element to monitor, it is important to know that depression can also be caused by poor nutrition.

REMEDIES TO ALLEVIATE DEPRESSION

Usually, the first suggestion I make to someone in an unhappy or depressed state is to focus on getting up earlier each morning and then walk or do some other form of exercise for a minimum of twenty-five minutes to increase the breath. The "runner's high" happens after twenty-five minutes of running or jogging, when feel-good hormones called *endorphins* are released in the body after a sustained increase in physical activity. Because endorphins create a sense of well-being, they can help alter feelings of negativity and depression; it then is easier for someone to produce more positive thoughts and have more clarity, which in turn lead to feelings of greater happiness.

I cannot diagnose or prescribe, but I often counsel my depressed clients to consider taking a supplement of some kind that can both help to lift one out of misery and change the chemistry in the body. Research shows that St. John's Wort can work as effectively as pharmaceutical drugs, and many people feel better after taking it partly because serotonin levels rise; this also happens with GABA (gamma aminobutyric acid) and 5-HTP supplements. Clinical studies have shown GABA helps to increase the production of alpha brain waves to create a sense of physical relaxation. The supplement 5-HTP promotes a calm and relaxed mood. It is a plant-derived amino acid that naturally increases the body's level of serotonin. Serotonin is made mostly in the gut but is utilized by the brain to achieve a sense of well-being. These supplements can also help ease what is known as "brain fog," or the inability to think clearly, which is one of the signs of depression.

Heather Tick writes about the importance of serotonin and other brain chemicals made in the gut and alludes to the importance of paying attention to your feelings: "The gut has 100 million neurons, or nerve cells—enough for a small brain. It produces 80 percent of our melatonin, which we used to think came only from the pineal gland in the brain, and it produces 80 percent of our serotonin, which is supposed to be the brain chemical that improves our mood. Why does our gut make chemicals associated with brain function? We don't yet really know, but maybe it explains why we have 'gut feelings.'"[2]

A CLIENT CASE EXAMPLE

The following case history illustrates depressive challenges as well as treatment interventions. I started working with Julia when she had just been diagnosed with recurring cancer near her groin. She had previously endured surgery, chemotherapy, and radiation and was having severe anxiety. I have learned through the years, both from the depression I had when I was younger and through my intuitive skills, to perceive signs of depression, such as the fear and desperation and tremors I heard, or rather sensed, psychically in Julia's voice. When she disclosed that she had insomnia and worry, felt unable to move forward, and did not know how to proceed, I knew she was moderately to severely depressed.

She was gasping for air as she talked; her words were tumbling over themselves. As she disclosed more about her financial situation and other issues that would play some role in her illness, I sensed more and more the signs of depression. Anxiety ran rampant through her voice and energy field. I knew it was important for her to calm herself and suggested that she think of something that made her feel peaceful. I also suggested she breathe slowly and deeply. It took several minutes for her to become calm enough so that we could chart a plan for recovery. I saw that it was possible for Julia to reverse the cancer and asked her if she could follow some positive-thought advice and do visualizations. She acknowledged that she would "try anything," and so we began.

We met weekly by phone, and I used quantum energy healing on the trouble spots in her body. At my suggestion, she also began recording her positive thoughts in a journal and doing self-forgiveness work, which is essential, as forgiveness of self and then others clears blockages so that energies can flow more easily. I encouraged

Julia to begin eating a healthier diet. She started eating more fresh vegetables and fruits and supplemented with nutrients suggested by her naturopath. Then, out of the blue, she received a shock: her supervisor told her she would lose her job and health insurance in two months, as the company was downsizing.

Two weeks later I knew Julia was in serious trouble, and not only with a return to ill health and in a deeper depression than I had noticed in our first few appointments. She had also lost her will to try to be healthier, she could not sleep, she did not want to eat, and she was so weak that she said she just wanted "to get it over with," which meant letting the cancer win.

As I would do with any client, I did my very best to help Julia turn herself around. I gave her positive suggestions and asked her to call in family to help with finances and loving support, and I encouraged her to prepare for her own personal downsizing. I suggested that she find a support group, a positive-thought community church, and reference material that would give her the information I thought she needed to turn the depression around. Her naturopathic physician cooperated by prescribing St. John's Wort, GABA, and 5-HTP to increase serotonin, as well as some excellent vitamins. She also recommended IV injections of vitamin C.

We worked through all of the issues that had surfaced with Julia's cancer and deep depression; little by little, I saw a shift take place as she began to make positive changes in her life. She found a support group and became creative in preparing healthy meals. I knew we were on the verge of success when she excitedly left me a voicemail message saying her latest tests had shown that the cancer was shrinking.

I intuitively knew that Julia would return to full recovery if she stayed on track with her positive thinking and the other changes.

Later I received a note from her. It had been a few months since she decided she would be fine on her own, with no further need of my intuitive or healing abilities. Her letter told me that her last scans showed that she was cancer-free and that she had returned to living a healthy life. She ended by saying how happy she had become.

Julia's case shows that anyone can heal from depression as well as serious physical conditions. Sometimes it just takes words of encouragement and, as in this case, a willingness and commitment to make positive lifestyle changes in order to overcome what may seem to be huge obstacles.

12

Beyond Ego, Forgiveness, and the Power of Ease

If instead of thinking *about Nature—identifying ourselves as a creation or product* outside *Nature—we allow ourselves to* feel *its soul running through us, then we find peace unfolding in our hearts and the unending wisdom of Nature's processes revealing themselves in our awareness.*

—RALPH WALDO EMERSON, *Natural Abundance*

These days, it is increasingly common to hear of research substantiating the benefits of healing touch and energy medicine. Recently, researchers at the University of California, Irvine, discovered that recovery for stroke patients who receive touch from caregivers is remarkable compared to the progress of those who are not touched and instead are only given standard drug treatments.[1] Practitioners in the art of transferring healing energy—whether through prayer, focused thought, or hands-on healing—may be interested in the technique.

FOCUSED INTENT TO HELP

There are many methods for the transfer of healing energy to others, but the basis of them all is a focused intent to help the other heal. That focus is the core of my practice. It is a key reason for the oftentimes remarkable healings that occur with my clients when they, too, have a strong intent to heal. There is a quantum jump into a realm of infinite and powerful healing energy when two or more join together in focused agreement for the purpose of prayer or healing.

RELEASING NEGATIVE ENERGY POSITIVELY AFFECTS THE BODY

Everything physical is, at its foundation, made of energy, and energy can be altered through intent. The following story is a wonderful example of the power of focused intent to align with the realm of healing energy in thought and feeling. A client named Gene, whose comments I quoted in a previous chapter, telephoned me with a concern. He said that a mole on his arm had grown from a very tiny spot to about the size of the head of a thumbtack within a two-week period, and he wanted my help. I intuitively saw what he was describing, which appeared to me as an elevated bump with "extra cells," reminiscent of cancer cells. I asked him to put his finger on the mole and to imagine my finger superimposed on his. He said he could feel the energetic presence of my finger, and after a short while, I told him that I now saw that the energy of the mole was gone, although its physical form still remained.

He said he could feel a shift in his emotions from worry to hope; he felt the desire he had that the energy of the mole had changed. Such feelings are subtle, but they are an important part of the healing process. I know Gene well, as we have worked together a number of times over a six-year period, and I have seen the strength of his intention that the power of energy medicine will work—indeed, it has worked for him many times. So it did not surprise me to hear, about two weeks later, that the mole had considerably decreased in size. Four months later, there was not even the slightest remnant of what had once been a fast-growing mole.

This healing technique I use is very simple. I basically visualize a healed condition and simultaneously send focused healing energy to the client. This has to be accompanied by the client's intent to accept healing. When both the healer and the client are open to the flow of healing energy, the conduit to the Source of all healing becomes greater. That is the reality behind the statement, "Wherever two or more are gathered in my name, there I am."

THOUGHT AND EMOTION AS BLOCKAGES TO HEALING

As I mentioned earlier, much dis-ease is caused by emotions and thoughts that block the natural flow of universal energy to our bodies. Many conditions that manifest in the body, such as heart dis-ease, cancer, fibromyalgia, and sinus pains, can be seen as emotionally based. These things can occur because the person wants to avoid doing something such as managing a certain stress or letting go of a particular self-image (for example, the concept that one is special because of an illness of some kind). I am reminded of JaneAusten's description of a character in one of her novels: "She is a poor Honey—the sort of woman who gives me the idea of being determined never to be well—& who likes her spasms & nervousness & the consequence they give her, better than anything else."[2]

Dis-eases can occur from holding on to habitual negative thoughts that prevent the body from receiving the natural and constant stream of well-being. When he asked for my help in eradicating a toenail fungus, Gene presented me with an example of how holding onto thoughts can affect the body. This is the type of issue that could easily be seen as physically caused but, as it turned out, had an emotional component that stemmed from an old, negative belief that he held.

Gene had been trying for ten years to eradicate a toenail fungus, which he thought might have come from wearing wet athletic shoes. He used to wade through streams while hiking and wear the wet shoes for miles; sometimes he soaked in natural hot springs. He said he had tried just about every remedy he could think of and asked me to help him heal with energy medicine, which I agreed to do. However, as I began to channel healing energy to him, I intuitively saw that there was more to the story, that the problem had either an energetic or emotional component.

As we talked, Gene recalled a long-forgotten memory that all of a sudden came to him. He remembered a scene from thirty years before, in which a young woman he had admired made the critical comment that his feet were too long. I noticed, as he said this, that he had taken that criticism to heart and never released it. I intuitively saw that Gene had been so embarrassed by the criticism that he had immediately begun judging his feet and toes and continued to do so for all these years. The negative thought had set up a holding area for a dis-ease process to begin.

Nothing he had tried served to eradicate the fungus, as that negative emotion was still living within him and negatively affecting his feet. I knew that he needed to shift this energy if there was to be a healing. We talked about how he could begin to appreciate his feet as beautiful—after all, one negative comment from someone who was out of alignment is not a reason to think negatively of one's body. Gene acknowledged that he had been subconsciously carrying this negative comment around with him for thirty years.

FINDING SOMETHING TO APPRECIATE

In a case such as Gene's, finding something to appreciate is quite important. The energy of appreciation is a high-frequency vibration. Whenever you appreciate—whether it is a person or thing that you love, the blue sky, your body itself, or life in general, the energetic frequency of your body rises. The light waves that are the basis of all physical matter and the substrate of molecules, DNA, and cells increase in power when there is appreciation. Appreciation allows well-being to flow naturally and facilitate the processing of old, diseased cells out of the body.

I encouraged Gene to appreciate his feet for all they had done to serve him, as this would be the basis for the beginning of the healing. Then I suggested that he reconstruct the original situation from a position of appreciation for his general health and his wonderful feet. Gene then visualized the person who had made the negative comment and imagined responding to her from his sense of appreciation and esteem of himself. He then told me he remembered that she had been in a negative mood; she was definitely not close to feeling appreciation when she criticized his feet. He imagined her as a little child when she spoke, and then he imagined a new response, one he would have said to a child: "Well, thank you for your opinion, but I think I have perfect feet just the way they are." Our cells, and even our DNA, can be changed in this way; this is self-healing.

As Gene went through this process, I continued sending healing energy to his feet, seeing them in a healed condition. After this session took place, Gene's toes had been doing much better—energetically, they were healed—but the fungus in the toenails took a bit longer to completely clear up as the nails grew out clean and healthy. There was an emotional healing, and this was followed by physical change for the better. There is really no dis-ease condition that cannot be reversed in this way.

Basically, what Gene did was to envision the past criticism from the woman as if it had happened in present time, and then he intentionally changed his thought about the original event in order to release the dis-ease state energy. In other words, he reframed the incident by imagining a new response to her criticism. "I like my feet the way they are," he said, and feeling the truth of that statement brought a smile to his face. I could hear it in his voice.

He also forgave himself for having ever thought otherwise, which involved aligning himself to his new view of his feet as being quite good-looking. If you have memories of negative events such as Gene had, you can work toward healing yourself by letting them go and forgiving yourself for having carried them around. It is very important to forgive yourself, to align to what you want and can appreciate, because it raises your vibratory frequency, which allows the full flow of well-being.

REFRAIN FROM JUDGING AND BE IN EASE

It is important to refrain from judging any part of your body; rather, love it all as perfect. After you see yourself as perfect, you can see others that way. We are all different but perfect. After releasing your judgments, all of which block the flow of energy, you will find it is far easier to be well than to be in dis-ease.

Thoughts of appreciation and self-love invigorate your DNA, so unhealthy cells, which are no longer welcome in your body, begin to disintegrate. They begin to lift off the body, allowing the space for healthy cells to replace them. In most of my healing sessions, I guide my clients through a process similar to this—lifting off the old cells and bringing in trillions of new, healthy ones.

Working with a healer can be much more effective than working alone because, as previously mentioned, when two or more are gathered for healing, the energy takes a quantum leap.

This all might seem mystical, but it is important to remember that many scientists are quietly becoming modern mystics because their findings prove the existence of a powerful source of well-being. Quantum physicists such as Amit Goswami speak to the connectivity between our bodies and consciousness as a whole and stress how important it is to create a world of solutions to the problems we might have. Goswami states that our challenge is to move beyond ego mode to the more powerful expanded quantum consciousness that is a part of us.

This is the realm from which the fountain of well-being flows to us. Goswami asserts, "Actually, we [scientists] have done our job. The scientific evidence for spirituality that includes experimental data is already here. My question to you is: 'What are you doing about it?'"[3]

What we can do to achieve optimum health is to be in ease and allow the flow of well-being, which is always there, underlying all we can see. We can take the time to examine our thoughts and emotions and make sure we are free of those that cause resistance and separation from this flow of well-being. We can also ask for help from healers of many kinds to assist us, and that includes those unseen angels whom we can access through prayer. All it takes is a little focused intent and practice to begin a journey of healing.

13

Our Bodies and the Profound Health Effects of Appreciation

Love is the perfect stillness and the greatest excitement, and most profound act, and the word almost as complete as His name. . . . One day He did not leave after kissing me.

—RABIA, in *Love Poems from God*

To appreciate is to love. The best way to love your body and soul is to appreciate them, to find something to appreciate. The body is so remarkable. It is not as solid as we thought. As physicist David Bohm and others have shown, physical matter is made of slowed-down light waves. Bohm and others working in the field of quantum physics throughout the twentieth century repeatedly noted that the body is not solid, but is, at the subatomic level, made of particles of energy that are also interrelated waves. It is important to remember this because it means any condition in the body, which is essentially made of wave energy, can be healed.

Theoretical physicists Bob Tolpen and Fred Alan Wolfe wrote, "The speculation that matter may be . . . trapped light energy arises from the famous Einstein formula $E=Mc^2$, which equates energy, *E*, and matter, *M*, by multiplying the latter by the speed of light, *c*, twice."[1] To Bohm and other scientists, it became clear that the body is not concrete; at the subatomic level of observation, physical matter is not solid.[2]

Physics researchers say that light energy is what structures matter; that is, "matter is organized through the interaction of molecules composed of slowed-down light."[3] How our minds and emotions, our consciousness, can influence our bodies is much easier to imagine in light of these findings of science. This is not a new way of looking at mind-body interaction. Almost one hundred years ago, physicist Sir Arthur Eddington asserted that our minds are preeminent over our bodies, which, though physical, are made of subatomic light waves and are therefore, at a certain level, non-solid. You could say that the subatomic waves are an effect of the stronger light of consciousness. Eddington wrote, "Recognizing that the physical world is entirely abstract and without 'actuality' apart from its linkage to consciousness, we restore consciousness to the fundamental position."[4]

HOW THE MIND CAN BENEFIT THE BODY

Our minds, thoughts, and feelings—our consciousness—can be seen as not only preeminent, but also as one with the body. This means that elements throughout the body, such as hormones and cells in the immune system and brain, are directly linked to one another and affected by consciousness. As National Institute of Mental Health neuroscience expert and biochemist Candace Pert notes, because of the immediate molecular interactions between our brains and bodies that occur with thoughts and feelings, researchers can no longer make a strong distinction between thoughts and the body with regard to hormonal and other chemical and molecular interactions and reactions.[5]

The bottom line here is that because consciousness is a preeminent determining factor in health, it behooves us to think well. Why? When you focus your conscious mind on something that feels good, something to appreciate, your body benefits profoundly. You not only feel good emotionally, but also, through thoughts and feelings that immediately affect the DNA and every cell in the body, you feel good physically. To continually think and feel appreciation is to facilitate an ever-present flow of well-being—which is love—thereby continually bathing the trillions of cells in your body in this flow.

It does not matter if you appreciate the smallest of things, such as the comfortable pillow on your bed or the fact that there is air to breathe; the effect is the same: feeling good. When you find something to appreciate about others with whom you interact, it does not matter if you can find only one thing. It is the focus that matters. Focusing on what feels good communicates to your DNA, which thrives best on appreciation.

The next chapter relates a healing story that incorporates all of these elements: the power of thought and intent, the non-solidity of the body, the use of energy medicine to affect a positive healing outcome, and the importance of the commitment to being fully healthy.

14

Healing Cancer with Energy Medicine

Spiritual is stronger than material force—thoughts rule the world.

—RALPH WALDO EMERSON, *Self-Reliance and Other Essays*

The following is a story from a man named Henry. It is about healing a skin cancer, which a dermatologist had diagnosed as basal cell carcinoma many years before. This story incorporates many of the principles of healing I have discussed so far, and a few new ones. Here is Henry's story as he wrote it to tell others:

"This particular dermatologist was interested in complementary medicine," my client began, "and she agreed with me that I could try to heal the minor skin cancer with natural treatments. However, through the years, despite these treatments, the irritation had endured and then begun to worsen. The skin cancer was near my right temple. Stress or sunlight would aggravate the skin condition, but I think the main factor was stress, as I was not managing it very well. The skin condition would become more red and itchy. I covered this spot for protection whenever I was in the sun.

"I was talking with Shannon McRae one day. We had moved to the town where she and her husband, David, lived, and I took the opportunity on a social occasion to ask her what she thought of the skin condition. I knew she could see energies underlying dis-ease and that she performed energy medicine healings. Unexpectedly, I heard her tell me that she thought I was pushing the envelope and I had better see a dermatologist. I immediately became more anxious but was hesitant to ask her for a healing session, thinking that, since she hadn't offered, it was beyond her skills.

"I made an appointment with a local dermatologist for mid-May, but I did not really want surgery unless I had explored and tried all known natural options. By now, the reddened area around what had been for years a small (.25 cm) skin cancer had grown to about the size of a half-dollar because of an allergic reaction to an otherwise effective glycol-nutrient cream I was using that contained an eggplant extract. I did not know at the time that I was allergic to nightshade vegetables like eggplants. Despite the increased reddening, I felt some comfort knowing I was going to see a dermatologist for treatment soon; on the other hand, I had not wanted my skin to be cut, so I increased my efforts to heal.

"The dermatology appointment was a month away. During that month I focused even more than usual on healing and wellness visualizations. For the three months prior, I had been focusing on the use of natural options—massage, reflexology, rebounding, meditation, craniosacral therapy, hydrotherapy, sunlight therapy, walking barefoot to connect to earth healing energies, and combinations of food nutrients and supplements—to make my body immunologically stronger. But, after Shannon's advice to see a dermatologist, I began to use even more natural remedies that could boost the immune system and flush out toxins, including Ojibwa (Essiac) tea. I focused, too, on using only the best, most live foods, and I began using a lot more antioxidant foods (berries, grapes) and supplements, including at least one milligram of selenium a day, along with the basics: vitamins A, C, and E in all the natural forms; probiotics; alpha-lipoic acid; chlorella and wheatgrass for cleansing; certain amino acids; and the Ojibwa tea for detox."

POWER OF INTENT TO FEEL COMPLETELY HEALTHY DESPITE CONDITIONS

Henry went on to describe what he did next: "In hindsight, probably the most significant thing I did—perhaps the *sine qua non* of all healing—was to begin decreasing my stress by using thought and feeling in a more focused way. I believed the condition was reversible, healable. I practiced freeing myself of negative emotions, intentionally investigating my past, and remembering painful moments that I could release or forgive myself for. Then I would practice the Emotional Freedom Technique to release the feelings of dis-ease from my emotions and body. I also read the book *DreamHealer*, by Adam McLeod, cover to cover and began practicing some of the methods Adam uses to heal others, such as seeing one's body, in a holographic form, as completely healthy, energetically.

"Adam's methods reminded me of Dora Kunz and her work in founding, along with Dolores Krieger, the Therapeutic Touch movement for doctors and nurses. I had worked with Dora for seven years in the late '70s and early '80s and had trained with her in her healing methods for two years. I also trained with other healers such as Alex Orbito from the Philippines, who does spiritual healing. I thought I knew a lot about energetic healings, but it is one thing to know and another to put the knowledge to use for oneself. Now I had to walk my talk, to practice what I preached about everything I had been learning in nutrition and mind-body health.

"One day, shortly after I had made the appointment with the dermatologist, I was talking with a good friend about the subject of total health and noted that we can be totally healthy. Adam and other faith healers could help heal people who participated in their own healing by visualizing themselves as whole. The healers would assist by seeing the body as a totally well hologram. The person with dis-ease focused on letting go of illness. Can't we each be healed in ourselves as well, if we practice it often enough?

"I also recalled the many cases I had heard or read about, such as those in Bernie Siegel's and Larry Dossey's books, and cases I had even witnessed myself with regard to spontaneous healings. Why not me? My friend then asked a crucial question: 'What will you do when you are totally well? How will you be?' And that stunned me, because I realized I had not let go of my sense that my body had dis-ease. I had become comfortable with uncomfortable situations. I was not envisioning how I would be with total wellness."

DIS-EASE AS A FRIEND

Henry had made an important discovery. He went on: "Curiously, when I examined my thoughts, I found I had not fully and completely believed that any of the remedies I was using would work. Had the condition really become such a friend that I was actually holding onto it? Was I attached to it as a sort of badge, making me special, giving me something unique to have to do? Is illness that which, as a powerless child, I used to get my needs for rest and attention met by the powerful parent? Had I brought that habit into adulthood? Was I staying committed to a current condition, no matter how uncomfortable, by identifying myself with ailing aspects of my past self? I found myself arranging and predetermining who I would be tomorrow based on those previous circumstances when, really, I wanted to change some or all of them. I would say, 'I have this illness,' as though it was a possession; such a statement is subtle, but it is a message to the subconscious self.

"Once I realized what was happening, I formed a strong intent to say and feel, 'I see evidence of this condition; it is from the past, but I hereby heartily focus on a feeling of improvement now, even if I can't see it.' I began to focus, 100 percent, on a new life story. Shannon had said, 'We often create barriers to a natural state of health and healing by not knowing what else to do.' Not knowing what it is like to be totally healthy, however, does not need to keep us from pre-paving each day as though we are completely healthy and really feeling it. It is very important to feel as though you are healthy, much the same way you might imagine feeling yourself lying on a beach in Hawaii as a way to inspire yourself to take a vacation there. You can actually feel the sun and the sand and the warmth, and then it becomes your eventual reality. The body does not know the difference between the actual sand and sun and the imagination and felt sense of it."

ARE YOU READY TO LET GO?

Henry and I finally started working together: "I made a decision to surrender, to set aside my sense of self-importance, and ask Shannon for an appointment to conduct a healing session. One evening, I remember it was May 2, she came over for a chat with my wife and me. I asked to schedule a healing for sometime soon, and she agreed. During a lull in our conversation, Shannon asked if I was ready for a healing. She said her arms and hands had begun getting warm, a sign to her that a healing was beginning; she said she felt energy starting to move through her and come toward me. I said that I was ready, even though it surprised me (delightfully) that she would do the healing session that evening. 'Are you ready to let go of the condition?' she asked, looking into my eyes.

"That was the essential question, and I knew I could not say yes unless I had complete integrity in saying so. Otherwise, it would be a waste of time. Shannon is very direct in a gentle, nonjudgmental way, and I loved this unconditional approach from her, a masterful psychologist who is also a medical intuitive and healer. When she asked, I immediately saw a challenge arise in my mind: letting go of a known thing, a condition, that had been a part of my way of being for more than ten years. Yet I knew that if I wanted the healing, I had the responsibility to let go or the healing would not happen regardless of what Shannon did; I knew at that moment I had to change my identity to that of someone who has no dis-ease and open myself to experimenting with life as a totally well person. It was a turning point.

"I not only said 'I'm willing to let go,' I also felt it deep within my soul, and at that moment, I recommitted myself to being in a new way, without dis-ease, no matter what changes would come into my life. I had prepared myself for this shift, though the opportunity to let go when Shannon asked, 'Are you ready to let go of the condition?' still perturbed me. But then a thought came to me: this is my life. So I decided to commit to the adventure of change. You have to feel good about feeling good in order to feel good as you move through the unknown changes."

SURRENDER AND HEALING INTENT

Henry had experienced a profound change and was ready for healing. "I had asked for a healing, and now I had to open to receive it by letting go of anything that would be a blockage. I surrendered, and Shannon started the healing energy, describing what she was seeing. As she did, I aligned to well-being and felt a wonderful wholeness in myself. I consciously intended to feel in surrender to the wholeness of well-being. I felt the surrender, and part of the reason I did is because Shannon was there in that same space, holding it with me. This is what a true healer does all the time: exist in the energy of well-being for healing.

"Shannon described how she felt the healing energy moving through her arm and hand and going to the spot on the side of my face. It was as though the energy was being directed by some unseen, conscious force. She described the process, saying that the energy appeared as a line of light, and she asked if I could feel it. I told her I could feel a tingling surrounding the spot and that I also felt a healing was taking place. There was a power that was palpable.

"Shannon said, 'Now I see this light has formed a concave shape completely under your skin. The first somewhat thin layer of the light is green; the second layer is lavender; and the rest of the concave area these colors define is filled with white light—energy. The white light is pulling negative energy out of the area and transmuting it into alignment with the universal light.'

"As she said this, I continued my focus on letting go of the cancer cells, feeling a very pleasant tingling sensation throughout the area surrounding the spot on my skin. I also felt as though I was in a different reality. It was very subtle, magical. At this point I was looking at Shannon, and she said that she saw my face disappear and turn into light. It felt as though time stopped at that instant. It seemed as though I moved into a parallel world during the healing, a world of wellness. Indeed, my world would have to change in order for me to move into physical wellness from a condition of dis-ease."

ARE YOU READY TO ACCEPT YOUR HEALING?

Henry was so ready to be healed at this point. He went on: "A minute later Shannon said the healing had occurred. She asked, 'Are you ready to accept your healing?' She awaited my answer. I was challenged. I knew a healing had occurred—I knew this was a turning point, an opportunity—but I had not expected her question, and it challenged my commitment again.

"I looked within my feelings and thoughts and said, 'I accept the healing.' I truly felt the honesty of it. I was also sure that being in this new way would bring its challenges, and I consciously decided to take on the challenges with joy and courage. Shannon smiled when I answered 'yes'; it is more accurate to say she was delighted. My wife had been participating by sitting silently by in harmony with the healing; we all wished each other a good evening, and Shannon departed.

"About ten minutes later I was preparing for sleep for the night. I turned on the light in the bathroom, looked in the mirror, and saw that the reddened area on the side of my face had puffed up at least an eighth of an inch. It was tingling a bit, and not only that, but light yellowish beads of moisture were appearing on the surface of the puffed area. The area was about the same size it had been for the past week, ever since the allergic reaction, but now it was puffed up instead of smooth.

I wiped off the moist beads with a tissue and observed the area. Had I not heard of 'healing crisis,' I might have been alarmed at what appeared, on the surface, to be a worsening of the irritation. However, I determined that this new condition represented the healing as well as the letting go I had done emotionally and mentally; along with my emotional letting go, my body was releasing cancer cells and whatever else was in the area, such as the allergens from the topical treatments I had used. I wiped more beads of moisture from the area ten minutes later and went to bed, focused on being in full health.

"When I looked in the mirror the next morning, I saw that there was no swelling and the redness had decreased. Now my intent, stronger than ever, was to have the area be totally healed by my appointment with the dermatologist in two weeks. I did not want the doctor to say that something was wrong and that I needed surgery or radiation or drugs.

"During that time, I practiced reaching for the feeling of total well-being. It was a new way of being. I would do what I had to do each day, taking care of necessary details, and then I would do what I found joy in doing, including my journal work or even rest, whereas before, I would continue to push myself to do more. I experienced, in a new way, the creativity of aligning with well-being, and I appreciated the big and little things: the earth spinning in its orbit, the food that is so abundant, the amazing well-being that keeps all our bodies going."

YOU HAVE NOTHING TO WORRY ABOUT

Henry was now experiencing the complete benefits of energy healing: "By the day before my dermatology appointment, the cancer seemed to have disappeared, and there was just a small area of slightly pink skin remaining. I passionately wished it would be gone before my appointment. Then, as if by coincidence, I received a phone call from the dermatologist's assistant later that day asking if I could postpone my appointment by five days!

"Five days later, even the pinkish area, where there had been deep redness and inflammation, had cleared up. The skin looked normal and healthy. The dermatologist introduced himself at our appointment and asked, 'Why are you here?' I said I was concerned that I might have had a non-healing skin cancer. He requested that I remove my shirt so he could examine me. I told him the history of the spot on my face and explained that it was not there anymore because, between the day I had made the original appointment and the day I showed up for it, a healer had helped me heal the area.

"Nevertheless, I wanted his diagnosis of the current state of the skin on my face. He stopped me as though he did not want to hear more of that story, put his glasses on, and observed the skin for a minute. He then took off his glasses, stood in front of me, looked into my eyes and said, 'My friend, you have nothing to worry about. There is nothing here but healthy skin. Go home and have a good day.'

"A few days later I asked Shannon to help me understand several details of the healing session. I wanted to know if she had ever undergone the same kind of experience with others who asked her for healing assistance as she had with me, where she saw a face 'disappear.'

"She became quiet and then replied, 'I started to experience that about twenty years ago.' I waited for more. 'I notice that when I do the healings, I access a timeless zone,' she continued. 'It seems I go into a place beyond time, and then that affects the one who wants the healing, too. I have noticed that when I am face to face with someone who is ready to change, the healing occurs simultaneously with the person's physical face "disappearing" in front of my eyes. It is as if the person has agreed to enter this different world, where healing always exists for all of us. When I do not see this disappearance, I know the person is not willing to enter the zone or receive the healing, because it is an individual's agreement to change to a healed state that is part of the cause of the disappearing face.'

"It is now close to six years since the dermatologist's finding: 'you have nothing to worry about.' Friends have asked to see the place that had been occupied by a skin cancer, and they are delighted by what they see, which is normal, healthy skin.

"Shannon told me, 'Many of us don't know what it feels like to be fully well, so we fear it.' It is new and is much like learning to ride a bicycle for the first time. Yet we know we are worthy of total well-being. We need only do everything we know in the current moment to be healthy, including just being in ease and resting, if need be. We need emotional freedom from dis-ease each moment.

"But as Shannon and other healers have noted, often we feel a sense of self-importance and get some kind of attention, either from self or others, because of our dis-eases. I now realize it is far easier and more joyful to be well. We just have to decide that we are going to feel better each minute and start the journey of leaving behind what does not feel good.

"Shannon also told me, 'We often adopt beliefs about things that we think can affect us, such as the flu. Then we look for evidence to validate the belief, such as slight feelings of illness or news that flu is overtaking the community.' One can begin healing by making peace with where one is, forgiving, and saying, as those who practice the Emotional Freedom Technique do, 'Despite all conditions such as the feeling of flu or negative past events, I deeply love and completely accept myself now,' and this helps considerably, beyond the conditions, to begin the process of releasing any dis-ease. You then have to stay focused on where you want to arrive on your journey, and you will get there.

"This is like driving from your house to the grocery story. Just because you are only halfway there, you don't get discouraged and say, 'Well, I'm not there yet,' and then turn around and go back. You just keep driving until you get there. Your desire is important and is akin to saying, 'Ask and you will receive.' Intend, stay focused, and you will be rewarded. The body just takes a bit of time to catch up sometimes, that's all, just like your auto journey to the store takes a while, but getting to the store is so rewarding."

THE MECHANICS OF HEALING

This process was a profound experience, for Henry as well as myself, and it clearly speaks to the power of focus and energy. My take on some of the mechanics of how healing takes place has to do with how a single particle of the body acts as if it is connected to other particles beyond space and time and is not limited by many of the laws science has constructed. When consciousness expands beyond limiting beliefs, we take the stuff we are made of and expand it, too. Our consciousness is that powerful. Max Planck, who is called the father of quantum theory, wrote, "I can tell you as a result of my research about the atoms this much: There is no matter as such! All matter originates and exists only by virtue of a force, which brings the particles of an atom to vibration and holds this most minute solar system of the atom together. . . . We must assume behind this force the existence of a conscious and intelligent Mind. This Mind is the matrix of all matter."[1] Scientific experiments have shown that, through the connecting fabric of the universe, our observations directly affect all waves and particles—especially those in our bodies.

15

Being Unconditionally Present as Part of the Healing Process

Love. You are forbidden to do anything other than that.

—BILL TOMES, in *Bridge between Worlds*

Many years ago I had the great pleasure of meeting and chatting with Elisabeth Kübler-Ross. She was a psychiatrist who was born in Switzerland and who was on the forefront of near-death experience research. She was instrumental in bringing hospice care to the United States in the mid-1970s. Her book *On Death and Dying* is popular with thousands of hospice medical doctors, nurses, case managers, and volunteers, as it helps them understand what terminal illness really means and how best to treat and help people who are reaching the end of their lives. Because of Kübler-Ross's work and the compassionate way she presented what she was doing with hospice through education, seminars, and speaking engagements, I was compelled to become a hospice volunteer, and worked as one for almost seventeen years. During that time, I learned more about the dying process than I would ever learn in my training as a psychologist.

LIFE STORIES AND RESOLVING ISSUES

Elisabeth Kübler-Ross had learned how best to meet people where they were when they were at a crossroads in their lives. She had found that she could not necessarily use her previous professional training with people who were facing death, so she developed ways to unconditionally support them in their heartfelt desires whatever those may be, such as resolving family or other relationship issues. In spite of the fact that many patients carried guilt and regrets, she found that all of them had wonderful stories to tell about their lives when she could just be there and listen. When telling their stories, they would light up and often find resolution.

These skills are equally valuable in working with clients who are not in a near-death situation. What I learned from my years in hospice is that the most powerful ways I can help as a therapist and medical intuitive is to be unconditionally present and listen and support others in their goals, which might be to heal a physical, mental, or emotional condition. The last chapter in this book speaks directly to death and dying issues as well as what I know to be life after death. For now it will suffice to say that often during the dying process issues can arise from unresolved relationship issues with family members, a spouse, or other people in the person's life, and so many times, just listening and tuning in enables me to help them resolve these issues.

NONJUDGMENTAL LISTENING AND INTUITION

One example of how nonjudgmental listening works can be provided by the story of a call I received from Edna, a very distraught grandmother. She was concerned about her ten-year-old granddaughter,

Amy, whom she described as a sweet, creative, and artistic girl who was very giving toward others. Amy was in a hospital undergoing tests to find the cause of a terrible headache she had been suffering from for weeks. The brain scan showed a cyst at the top of her brain. Amy not only suffered from awful headaches, but her skin had also become pale and she could not carry out her usual activities. The doctors told Amy's parents and grandmother that they could not determine what to do, and they advised taking a wait-and-see attitude.

Edna said she knew of my intuitive energy healing work and that she had faith. I told her that the power of trust and faith between us must have a positive outcome, as in an answer to prayer. Edna agreed and asked me to begin long-distance healing work for herself as well as for Amy, which I did immediately. We planned to talk again in a few days, after I had had a chance to work in this way.

I called Edna at our appointed time a few days later, and she said Amy was still having headaches but was feeling more peaceful. During our conversation I received an intuitive insight: Amy's difficulty arose from a trip out of the country. I asked Edna to find out whether Amy had traveled to a foreign country in the past few years. Edna said she had, and in fact, their entire family had spent vacations in Mexico and other South American countries, where they often swam in rivers and the ocean. I then told her that I strongly suspected there was a parasitic cause to Amy's cyst and that Edna's disclosure that they had swum in the waters there confirmed it for me. Edna became excited and said that she herself had suffered a major bout with a parasitic infestation in her intestinal tract after one of their family vacations during which she had been swimming.

Hearing this, I felt even more strongly that I was correct about the parasite. I also felt relief, not only because I had once again received confirmation about the power of intuition, but also because it was helping to solve the puzzle of Amy's condition. After the phone call, I continued the healing energy work for Edna. Her intent was to be calm and more present in a balanced way for Amy and the rest of the family. At the beginning of the healing session, as I tuned in I could see that Edna was carrying enormous stress. I put myself in a place of peace and calm and then channeled that energy to Edna. I focused on sending this energy to her for ten minutes a day for several days. At the same time, I worked on the cyst in Amy's brain, visualizing it decreasing in size. I did this for twenty to thirty minutes a day for two weeks.

I knew that the cyst in Amy's brain was creating an emergency situation, but I did not want to alarm Edna by saying so. Because of the danger the cyst posed, I spent more time than usual sending healing energies and working with diminishing it. As each day passed, I could see the cyst decreasing in size.

Edna called me two weeks later and reported that Amy's headaches had gradually subsided in conjunction with each session of energy healing I did for her. Edna had also talked with her son, Amy's father, about the possible parasitic cause of Amy's cyst. The father conveyed this information to the doctors, who then called in a specialist. The specialist ordered another brain scan for Amy. This scan showed that the cyst was smaller than it had been two weeks earlier; nevertheless, the doctor prescribed some medication.

By the time of this last scan, Amy had begun feeling much better. Her headaches were completely gone, her complexion was no longer pale, and she was slowly returning to her usual activities. Since then, she has continued to grow stronger, and I am heartened to know that Amy will lead a wonderful life, sharing her sunny disposition everywhere she goes.

It seems so apparent to me that working together with Edna enabled the healing for Amy to take place so well. It was our intent for healing, as well as the knowledge that a greater Source was behind it all, that made the healing possible.

I have long felt my greatest purpose in life is to help others in their healing processes to the best of my ability. If I had not had my earlier hospice experiences with very critically ill people, I would not have gained the presence of mind, faith, and trust to offer what I feel I can do to be of help. Also, my experience as a therapist and my intuitive abilities are not so very uncommon anymore. Such abilities are increasingly emerging among people today as they are more recognized and accepted. As astrophysicist Bernard Haisch asserts in his book *The Purpose-Guided Universe,* "All humans possess a capacity to intuitively perceive the true multifaceted nature of ourselves and the greater reality."[1]

16

Healing by Letting Go of Emotional Pain

> ***Our primary hunger is not for objects or the experiences they can provide, but for bliss and freedom. We are hungering for ecstasy and, ironically, ecstasy is an experience that requires emptiness. It calls for letting go rather than acquiring.***
>
> —**BELINDA GORE,** ***The Ecstatic Experience***

All of us have emotions, and all of our emotions affect our physical bodies in some way. As I mentioned earlier, scientists such as Candace Pert have proven that emotions affect molecules in our bodies. [1] When someone is suffering ill health, the cause often seems to be a mystery. In such cases, intuitive medicine can be the most direct route to discovering causal factors in dis-ease.

Every human being has the ability to use the innate function we generally call intuition. However, there are those among us who have, for various reasons, focused on using this sense more than others have. It could be, as in my case, that there is trauma in someone's background that called for them to be super-sensitively aware of those around them in order to be forewarned of potential harm; or it might be that someone was raised by parents who were aware of this sense and did not dissuade them from it and even encouraged its use.

SUPER-SENSORY FOCUS

When someone has long used what has variously been called a super-sensitive perceptual focus, it becomes a natural part of life. Most people actually use this sense occasionally without focusing much awareness on the fact. For example, with close relations, there is often a sense of knowing when someone is going to call or even knowing what someone is going to say.

The following case illustrates how intuition can be used to help another. Janet called me; she was very much oriented toward using her intellectual left brain more than her creative right-brain aspects. She did not disclose certain key things to me, but at one point in our counseling session, I had an important intuitive insight. This is how it unfolded.

SCANNING THE BODY WITH INTUITIVE INSIGHT

Janet said she had worked with a number of medical intuitives, naturopathic physicians, and nutritionists and that nobody had been able to help her with intestinal disorders she had had for a number of years. We spent the better part of her first appointment going over her history, and I took lengthy notes to make sure I had an accurate report of what she was telling me. Prior to the end of that first appointment, Janet told me I was the first person she had talked with who had answered some of her questions along the way. She wanted to know if she might have to live with her condition for the rest of her life, and she challenged me as to whether I thought I had the tools to help her.

I knew I needed to learn as much as I could about this woman's complicated health difficulties. Just before ending our phone appointment, I scanned her body by remote viewing. (Remember, I only do this when clients give their consent.) Scanning revealed to me what seemed to be an out-of-balance thyroid; a hiatal hernia; acid reflux; scarring of her esophagus; ulcerative colitis; and Sjogren's syndrome, an autoimmune dis-ease involving the abnormal production of extra antibodies that attack the glands and connective tissue. Sjogren's manifests itself as dry eyes, dry mouth, and internal dryness. Janet confirmed these symptoms, and then she told me I was the only person she had found who would listen to all of her concerns. She said she wanted to continue working with me.

Our second appointment focused on nutritional needs and how Janet was handling the medications prescribed by her medical doctor. I could see intuitively that she was rapidly losing her health. Since I could sense that she was not yet open to my healing energies, I suggested the nutritional supplements I would take if I were in her deteriorating condition. I also suggested that she ask for a blood test that could show various autoimmune dis-eases, because she had disclosed to me some classic symptoms that reminded me of lupus, rheumatoid arthritis, Reynaud's, and, as I mentioned before, Sjogren's syndrome.

TRUST AND SELF-DISCLOSURE

Janet was such a puzzle to me at first. I strongly sensed that her challenges had causal factors that she was not disclosing, so I asked her directly what it was she was blocking me from knowing about her. She then started to confess. She was addicted to chocolate candy bars and carbonated colas; she was hiding them from her husband, as well. She also told me that I was the first person she trusted on her way to health because she did not feel I was judging her "like the others had," and that was why she revealed the chocolate candy bar and cola issue. One never truly knows if a connection will take place with a new client, but when trust is present, the potential for healing is much greater.

Janet said that she and her husband were going on an extended vacation and she would not be able to keep in touch with me for a few months. We discussed ways that she could take care of herself while away from home and how to manage what we had already discovered about her body.

During the months of silence from Janet, I sometimes wondered if she would ever call again. She finally did, and we made an appointment. I was dismayed to learn that her health had severely deteriorated and none of the specialists and alternative health care practitioners she had seen while traveling had been able to figure out what was causing her decline. At my recommendation, Janet had a test that confirmed she did not have any autoimmune dis-eases, much to my relief. She said, however, that she could only eat five things and they made her stomach hurt, so it hurt almost all the time. She was so thin that her clothes hung on her. I paused to ponder this.

HEALING THE PAIN BODY

I had a sudden intuitive insight and asked Janet what had happened when she was between the ages of four and seven. She replied that she had rheumatic fever at age five, was home-schooled by her mother, and was in bed for months. "Aha," I thought, "we are on to something deeper!" Then I asked how her family treated her during this time and if she felt loved. Janet answered that she felt like a terrible burden to her family and had always felt guilty for being so sick.

She revealed that after she got well, at about age eight, her mother took a picture of her in a pair of shorts to show her relatives how fat her legs had become; she had then been subjected to ridicule by her family about her fat legs during the years before she left home for college and marriage.

Knowing that I had found a key to helping Janet return to health, I very gently elicited from her what she had done with her feelings of guilt and lack of self-worth and her negative thoughts. Slowly but surely she began to open up to me about her past, like a new flower about to bloom. As I usually do with all my clients, I had been holding a place of being fully present with her to hear and accept what she said without judgment. As she answered my questions, she opened to her own answers.

I could feel a rush of healing energy begin to swirl around and through her. I knew that she had turned a corner toward accepting health for her body and accepting her body as the carrier of healing energies. I could see that she would finally be able to forgive herself for accepting the negativity directed at her by others (knowing she had done so because of lack of knowledge). This forgiveness and acceptance of herself was also key to her forgiveness toward those who had not realized what they had put her through for so many years. Janet is on her way to complete health, and she has begun to see herself as a beautiful human being in a beautiful human body.

Janet's story gives a poignant example of what Eckhart Tolle calls the "pain body." Globally, more than 15 million people have heard Oprah Winfrey and Eckhart speaking about Eckhart's book *A New Earth* via Oprah's website. Briefly, a pain body is an emotional energy body that most of us create and often keep alive from early childhood by not resolving pain when it enters our lives. Let us look at the case of Janet's pain body.

When Janet was a child, her sense of feeling burdensome to others became a pain body. She became increasingly identified with this feeling, even though it was painful. She began to see others through the lens of this emotional baggage, and she acted and reacted based on it.

Unless you resolve the painful emotions and events in your life, you may become identified with this pain; your ego acclimates to the pain, identifies with it, and even becomes addicted to it. You begin to respond to others with fear or anger, and your response keeps feeding that pain body, enabling it to remain strong. The painful emotion produces correspondingly painful molecules in the physical body, and all sorts of physical conditions can result.

So many times in the course of using energy medicine, the trail we follow leads back to things that happened years ago; often, these painful events are still energetically stuck in the subconscious, influencing habits even if there is little memory of the actual events.

Janet found it difficult to remember events and circumstances that needed to be addressed in her healing process. However, she agreed to try, and with courage and determination she began the process of forgiveness—first learning to forgive herself, and then others. At her own pace, and with my encouragement each step of the way, she has realized progress. She is now able to eat a variety of foods that do not hurt her stomach, the hiatal hernia has been corrected, the acid reflux is at a minimum and her esophagus has healed nicely, and she has put aside her addiction to chocolate bars and colas. We occasionally have follow-up appointments, and Janet continues to improve not only her physical health, but also her diet and her attitudes and thoughts about people in her life. I can hear a new lilt to her voice that had not previously been present.

17

The Energies of Emotions and Their Effects on the Body

Look at everything as though you were seeing it either for the first or last time. Then your time on earth will be filled with glory.

—BETTY SMITH, *Joy in the Morning*

It is fascinating to perceive through intuition, as I do, the energetics of emotions and the physical body as well as how they interact with one another in both health and illness. Because I have had many experiences with physical illnesses myself beginning at an early age, I long ago developed a desire to use my intuitive knowledge and insights to assist others in healing themselves.

Scientific studies have begun to substantiate the efficacy of intuitive insight and energetic healing. For example, the Institute of Noetic Sciences (IONS) was founded in 1973 by former astronaut Edgar Mitchell for the purpose of conducting and sponsoring leading-edge research into the potentials and powers of various aspects of consciousness, including perceptions, beliefs, attention, intention, and intuition. (For more information, see www.noetic.org.) Many of the world's leading scientists are members or extended faculty of IONS. They include Richard Moss, Charles Tart, and Rupert Sheldrake. These and other scientists have for decades been studying "inner knowing," an intuitive awareness that gives direct and immediate access to knowledge beyond what is available to our normal senses. Their findings, along with the revelations of quantum physics—revealing that our physical bodies are not solid but are made of light waves—often describe the types of extrasensory perceptions I have had for many years.

A CASE IN POINT

Countless people have heard about my work because I have had so many successes in helping others heal. One such person is Jane, who called to present me with complaints about several conditions that she said were draining her energy; she mentioned insomnia, headaches, arthritis in her hands and elbows, colitis, and a bladder infection, as well as her belief that she was beginning to "fade away." She stated that she could hardly get outside and take a walk to her mailbox because she was so weak.

At Jane's request, I scanned her body over the phone. I do most of my work this way, as distance is no barrier to intuitive perception. I receive insights from the body itself, as if it reveals to me its state of health or dis-ease organ by organ, system by system. I perceived immediately that there were strong emotional and mental issues affecting Jane's physical body. As with other clients, some of my work involved interpreting energy patterns in and around Jane's energy fields, so I could determine what physical components might be out of balance due to unresolved emotions. This enabled me to begin to help correct her energy flow. It seems that the vast majority of physical ills stem from stressful thoughts that are repeated until they become beliefs, resulting in erratic emotions, as these invariably show up in the troubling of the body.

The main challenges for Jane were a fear that I (or any therapist) would drop her, a disinclination to follow any specific program leading to health (in body, mind, or spirit), and a need to create a commitment to heal herself. Her main physical ills were insomnia, a low-functioning thyroid and resultant lack of energy, and a very inflamed intestinal tract. Her low energy affected her ability to prepare nutritious foods and eat well; it also affected her ability to focus on healing.

I helped Jane implement a nutritional program that would begin to balance her intestinal tract and help heal it from the traumas of poor food choices. As I explained, she would have more energy available to help her thyroid heal and would have less insomnia if she was to follow this program. It was important she (and all of us in general) focus on an alkaline diet that included probiotics and digestive enzymes, all of which would help heal not only the colon, but also the whole body. I also suggested the more alkaline goat kefir and goat yogurt. (Goat milk is generally much more friendly to the human digestive system than cow milk.)

THE POWER OF INTENT

Jane began to make dietary changes with the intention of healing. I stress the factor of intention, because when there is chronic illness, healing cannot take place without intention. Sincere intent to be completely healthy can lead to powerful changes in one's energy fields, which in turn instruct the body. Lynne McTaggart is on the forefront of research showing that intention is crucial; she focuses on energy fields and has written extensively about them in her books *The Field* and *The Intention Experiment*. Her research shows that intentions are real and definite forces of energy that have demonstrable effects on the body. Thought and emotion are creative forces, and when we use them intentionally for exactly what we want, they do change our physical bodies, starting at the molecular level.

Jane's intention for better health gave her a feeling of trust in herself, and her intent had immediate effects on her energy field, which then started to influence her physical body. During our initial session, I used healing energy to give more strength to her body.

THYROID DYSFUNCTION FROM SELF-INHIBITION

It became apparent that Jane was often afraid to speak things that she knew to be true. This insight gave me a clue that her thyroid might be dysfunctional, which is very often the case when one chronically inhibits the power of speech. Indeed, as I looked at her thyroid energetically, I could see it was not functioning well. I suggested foods such as kelp, a small amount of iodized salt (although I do not recommend this except under extraordinary circumstances), and green, leafy vegetables to continue to help energize her thyroid. I also suggested she consider asking her complementary medicine physician about a liquid iodine supplement to help her thyroid.

Jane's insomnia had been out of control for a long time, so I suggested she begin to use a therapy such as Emotional Freedom Technique (EFT) to create relaxation for naps and a restful night's sleep. Also, if her doctor recommended it, she could take melatonin, a sleep enhancer made naturally in the body, for a short time to help her get a better quality of sleep and more strength in her overall energy fields.

EFT AND FORGIVENESS

During subsequent sessions Jane and I worked hard together, using EFT and practices relating to forgiveness (of self and others) as Jane attempted to gain insight into lack of self-worth. Self-forgiveness for not esteeming one's self in the past can be very powerful and can free one up to be in the moment, which, indeed, is just where health can be claimed most potently.

Sharing a little more of Jane's background will help to understand her case. Jane had very strict parents and felt that she never received approval for anything she accomplished. She experienced constant criticism from her parents and started overeating to fill her need for approval. Ultimately, she developed the pattern of judging herself for being overweight. She repeatedly thought of her overweight condition as being less than desirable, to the point that she formed the strong belief that she was flawed; then she constantly criticized herself for it. This belief showed up in her energy fields as emotional patterns of despair and curtailed expression of her true self, which became hidden beneath layers of low self-esteem.

I taught Jane to use EFT for her low self-esteem as well as for her insomnia and low thyroid functioning, which we learned were also related to her perception of herself as being overweight. EFT is excellent in that it is very simple yet quite effective in helping people who wish to release unwanted emotions. The EFT technique involves tapping certain acupuncture points on the head, face, and upper torso while focusing on specific types of statements that assist one in releasing the emotions that are no longer desired. Jane began by focusing on this statement: "Despite my overweight condition, and despite my judgment of myself, I am beginning to deeply love and completely accept myself."

In EFT, tapping on specific points is what releases emotions from the body, while forgiveness of oneself and others is what releases emotions from the energy fields. This procedure can be repeated for thirty days in order to stop the thought/emotion dis-ease pattern. Often, when an emotion is cleared, the related physical maladies disappear without drugs or surgery. It would be very beneficial if more medical doctors were to work directly with their patients to find out what emotional stresses are taking place.

Jane and I worked weekly for more than six months and were able to resolve her many issues so that, by the time we finished our sessions, Jane had confidence and healthy self-esteem to help her face a new life adventure of her choosing.

18

Coherence and Unexpected Healing

When you pet a dog or listen to a cat purring, thinking may subside for a moment and a space of stillness arises within you, a doorway into Being.

—ECKHART TOLLE, *Guardians of Being*

Kelly A. Turner, a consultant in the field of integrative oncology, focuses on case histories of the unexpected remission of cancer—"a remission," she writes, "that occurs either in the absence of Western medicine or after Western medicine has failed to achieve remission."[1]

Turner writes, "In the medical world, this kind of case is referred to as a *spontaneous remission,* which is defined as 'the disappearance, complete or incomplete, of cancer without medical treatment or with medical treatment that is considered inadequate to produce the resulting disappearance of disease symptoms or tumor.'[2] Many researchers, including myself, believe that the word *spontaneous* is a misnomer and should be changed to *unexpected* or *unlikely*. We feel this way because few things in life are truly spontaneous—occurring purely by accident. It is more likely that these remissions have a cause—or two or three—that science has not yet identified."[3]

Many in the healing profession have worked with untold numbers of clients who have had what Turner now calls unexpected remissions. It does not matter what we call them, says Turner. "Unexpected remissions do occur, and more than one thousand cases (across all types of cancer) have been published in medical journals. Thousands more have most likely occurred but not been published, because most doctors don't take the time to write up a report and submit it to a journal."[4]

THEMES IN SPONTANEOUS HEALINGS

In the late 1980s, the Institute of Noetic Sciences launched the Spontaneous Remission Project, which culminated in the publication of a comprehensive bibliography of documented cases.[5] After interviewing fifty non-allopathic healers who work with cancer patients and conducting seventy hour-long interviews with recovered patients, Turner isolated several "very frequent" treatments and three "strong beliefs" that both the patients and healers think helped to heal the subjects who had experienced unexpected healings.

Belief 1: Change the conditions under which cancer thrives. One of Turner's healer interviewees says, "The most successful recoveries seem to be strongly associated with major mental, emotional, or physical behavioral changes among the people with the illness."[6]

Belief 2: Illness is a blockage or a slowness in natural physical health, and health is associated with movement. The patients who healed believed that cancer represents a "blockage or slowness somewhere in the body-mind-spirit system, whereas health occurs when there is a state of unhindered movement or flow,"[7] or, as I believe, non-resistance to well-being in body, mind, and spirit.

Belief 3: The body, mind, and spirit are connected and interact with one another, and well-being can permeate all three of these levels of awareness. One of the healers said, "You have to have mind, body, and spirit healing. . . . Most of us who live in our physical bodies, we don't even know about spiritual or emotional bodies. So we have to connect with all three of them."[8]

There were four practices that the cancer survivors and healers focused on most frequently. The first was changing to a diet of primarily whole foods, such as vegetables, fruits, and grains, and eliminating alcohol, sugar, refined grains, and excess meat. They focused on more raw or slightly cooked foods and vegetable juices.

The second thing they did was to focus on deepening their feeling of a divine, loving energy by doing such things as meditating or contemplating quietly and alone many times during the day. One person who experienced an unexpected healing of cancer said that he could feel energy swirling around and through every cell in his body. This feeling of energy might be referred to as being in a state of coherence, which I discuss in the following section.

The third was to intentionally look for reasons to feel love, joy, and happiness in even the smallest details of their lives, and the fourth was to release repressed emotions such as fear, anger, and grief. One survivor had overcome pancreatic cancer; she said she believed it was an energy that was stuck in her body. I have found it to be the case that, for someone who has cancer, often there is some grief or fear or resentment that has not been resolved.

Those who healed also took herbs and vitamins to support the release of toxins and help the immune system; they used their intuition to help make treatment decisions; they took control of health decisions instead of passively accepting whatever their doctors told them; they said they had a strong will to live, defying any doctor telling them they had only two or five years to live; and they found social support from others, including other healers.

One correspondent responded to Turner's work by writing the following personal disclosures in the comment section that followed

Turner's article: "I thank you with all my heart for reporting on this possibility. I have heard it said that more people die from the [cancer] treatment . . . and that many physicians would decline the Western [medical] protocols [themselves]. As for me, I am following many of the recommendations . . . and expect to live many more years healthy and happy. I have discovered that spiritual healing is the most powerful."[9]

HEART INTELLIGENCE AND COHERENCE

Let us look at some of the factors that can play a role in the feelings that provide well-being and ultimately foster unexpected remissions. One way to discuss the feeling of well-being is to put it in the context of a feeling of coherence. Gregg Braden states that "while the brain is certainly important, it is not the first organ that forms in the body."[10]

Braden notes it is the human heart that forms first and that there is a scientific mystery about what triggers the first heartbeat. Science, he says, cannot so far tell us definitively why the heart starts to beat: "In one moment in time, there is a mass of cells, and then something happens and the heart starts to beat."[11]

Braden then notes something that is crucial to understand about the well-being of our bodies and their ability to heal: "As the [heart] develops, it begins to regulate the chemistry through the rest of the body. The heart sends the electrical signals to the brain that trigger the chemistry in the brain that is released to the body."[12] Then he says the chemistry that is triggered is based on the way we feel.

What we feel sends chemical signals throughout the body. Braden asserts, "The electrical signal between the heart and the brain is the key to understanding this relationship. When we are in what is called *coherence*, an experience that is measured as 0.10 Hz, 0.10

cycles per second, [or] when we are feeling the feelings that allow us to experience 0.10 cycles per second; that is when our coherence is optimum; that is when we are sending the optimum signal between our heart and our brain."[13]

Researchers at the Institute of HeartMath note that "personal coherence . . . refers to the synchronization of our physical, mental, and emotional systems. It can be measured by our heart-rhythm patterns: The more balanced and smooth they are, the more in sync, or coherent, we are. Stress levels recede, energy levels increase and our brain and what HeartMath calls the 'heart brain' are working together. It is a state of optimal clarity, perception and performance."[14]

The feelings that lead to coherence are those that come from positive focus: appreciation, peace, and finding joy in the moment. Coherence occurs when our brain begins to release unique chemistry into our bodies that effects healing, and one outcome is that our immune systems are invigorated. For example, the anti-aging hormone DHEA increases 100 percent over a three-minute period just from having positive feelings.

COHERENCE AND THE STABILITY OF OUR BODIES

Gregg Braden says, "In the presence of coherence, we become less aggressive, more peaceful."[15] What is coherence? Coherence, as it relates to our bodies, can be defined as the organizational stability of the molecules, cells, and all systems of the body. A coherent system operates as one unit. Our bodies are coherent systems made of cells, tissues, and organs, and they function as one unit. However, our bodies are also affected by our thoughts and feelings, for good or ill. Coherence occurs when we are completely aligned in thought and feeling with total health. Our cells are constantly aligning themselves to coherence.

It may be that there is a condition of illness in the body. By focusing one's thoughts and feelings on total health rather than on a condition that appears otherwise, coherence is brought to the body. The overriding well-being of coherence, or the feeling of it, is what brings faster healing, oftentimes unexpectedly. Coherence allows the cells in the body to stay organized, the system whole, and well-being intact.

It is interesting to note that seeing structures such as our global system, and even larger systems, as being in coherence despite outward appearances is also useful. Let us consider how coherence can help us see that consciousness outside the brain—the natural flow of well-being—is a fact.

We can easily understand that a more expanded part of ourselves, the mind, affects the brain. Our minds and the individual thoughts we think are inseparable from our feelings and bodies. Alignment in thought and feeling with the coherence of universal or natural well-being—outside any existing condition—creates feelings in the body that cause the brain, as Gregg Braden says, "to release life-affirming chemistry into our bodies."[16]

I have regularly experienced expanded, coherent consciousness most of my life. It is easy for me to explain such expanded awareness and how it can benefit anyone. It is also what I focus on in my work to help others heal. I can understand what is taking place in another's body, emotions, and sometimes thoughts because of the existence of expanded consciousness. I learned that the body follows thought by my own personal experiences and by using my intuitive insights to help others heal.

Consistent negative thought triggers negative emotion and belief. Over time, consistent negativity creates an imbalance in the body. Sick cells are really the manifestations of these imbalances. There is a lack of coherence because the negative thoughts and emotions are creating resistance to the overall natural flow of well-being to the cells. Here I again point out an important factor in reversing negative thinking: it is crucial to monitor our thoughts and to forgive ourselves for any negative ones because they can otherwise easily lead to accidents or other negative events, including physical illnesses.

SELF-FORGIVENESS AND COHERENCE: A CASE HISTORY

The following story is an example of not only how negative thoughts and emotions lead to physical problems, but also how coherence in mind, body, and emotion can bring unexpected healing. Wendy called me and presented a multitude of problems, including colitis. Her husband had just left her for another woman after two years of secret infidelity; he had also been physically abusing Wendy. She was in shock after he left her, and shortly thereafter she began to experience severe ulcerative colitis. She also received a diagnosis of early-stage breast cancer.

These conditions stemmed from the stress she felt due to her husband's infidelity. She also learned later that she had hepatitis B. Wendy did not want to follow the allopathic protocol her doctor outlined for any of these conditions and instead found a competent naturopathic physician, who began treating her with natural remedies and complementary medicine. She asked me to be part of her team; specifically, she wanted my help to resolve negative emotions in order to be at peace with the chaos around her and to help bring her body back to health.

I intuitively felt that it was possible for her to return to a normal state of health, but only if she was willing to gradually do forgiveness work, and she followed my suggestions about how to do so. Sometimes I can almost hear a groan from clients when I tell them a return to health involves their need to forgive themselves for all the negative thoughts and feelings they have harbored for any period of time, long or short. Often there is resistance. But when I explain that forgiveness will help to free up blockages in their emotions and bodies, they are willing to try it.

It was apparent to me that deep emotional pain had triggered this massive breakdown of tissue in Wendy's body. A person with conventionally oriented beliefs would think Wendy could not be expected to heal without drugs or other physical interventions, but she did heal without them. Here is what I think is the reason for her recovery.

Some of her pain and shock was very new and raw; we worked slowly and gradually in her forgiveness work so that she would not be further traumatized by focusing on too much at once. For example, we started out by barely touching the surface of what I saw as the underlying forgiveness process she needed to do, which was for deep negative thinking that was causing physical illness. I asked her about this, and she disclosed to me an excessively harsh self-sabotage message she continually repeated to herself. Wendy would repeatedly look back and judge herself harshly for not leaving her husband many years ago. Her son had told her many times she needed to leave him. So she had a very strong, chronic self-blame cycle going, which was the basis of her colitis.

Wendy's liver problems with the hepatitis B also stemmed

from this anger at her husband, herself, and her situation. She had imploded, in a way. She was self-destructing with her continual negative thinking. She was fearful and angry because she did not feel she could easily move away from her husband, yet she wanted to leave. Also, she learned she had contracted hepatitis B from her husband. He told her that he had contracted hepatitis B from his lover. Overall, Wendy could not seem to do what she needed to do regarding her own shortcomings and her insecurity.

Curiously, the breast cancer Wendy was experiencing was related to nurturing, but in a reverse way. She judged herself for not listening to her son's advice to leave her husband. Not following her son's urgings and continuing to stay in the marriage, even though it was very toxic, was an underlying factor affecting her breast issue, in that she was not nurturing herself. She began to do her forgiveness work immediately after our first session.

The process of forgiveness Wendy followed was gradual—to sincerely and continually respond to any negative thought that came to her mind by saying and feeling: "I am beginning to learn now to love and accept myself." She would also say and feel: "Despite the fact that I have not nurtured myself in the past, I now am learning to do so, and I am beginning to deeply love and completely accept myself."

When you feel deep love for yourself, which is always coming from Source, you heal. Again, when you think a negative thought, you pinch off this flow of love and well-being. When you forgive, you reopen to the flow. It is that simple.

I can say that after several months of working together with Wendy, and especially because of her forgiveness of herself, her ulcerative colitis disappeared and her hepatitis B reached a state of full remission. We made major inroads into her recovery from breast cancer as well, with energy medicine and forgiveness.

19

Intent, Focus, and Healing over a Long Distance

Positive Thought, Presence, and a Case of Healing the Lungs

> ***In time, as in space, the individual stretches out beyond the frontiers of his body.***
>
> **—ALEXIS CARRELL, *Voyage to Lourdes***

Author and doctor Larry Dossey has clearly shown that the effects of focused intent to send healing energy are not barred at all by space or time. (In fact, his book *Space, Time & Medicine* is a seminal work in this regard.) His research not only fascinates but also opens up many possibilities. In his book *Prayer is Good Medicine,* Dossey notes, "The vast majority of us pray, and believe our prayers are answered." He also writes, "There are different kinds of prayer, and evidence suggests that prayer, like drugs, can have effects that can be positive, neutral, or negative."[1]

Negative thought is clearly something that does not make us feel good. However, if we think positive thoughts such as "I can do this now" or "I expect a good outcome," or even a general thought such as "the sun came up today," we feel good. I know that in my healing work, I never focus on the negative or expect anything other than healing for a client who wishes it. I also know, from hundreds of successful experiences, that distance is not a barrier to focused healing intent as I, and others, use it.

Another example of such healing is Emily, who is 93. She had tripped on an outdoor mat and fallen down a cement staircase, and she could not get up. A neighbor who saw what happened immediately called 911. Emily was taken to a small local hospital, and after X-rays, the doctor said she might have a seriously injured spine. She was airlifted to a hospital in Seattle. The doctors took a CT scan and an MRI of her back and neck and determined that Emily's neck had been severely damaged; she was also quite bruised on various parts of her body. The doctors doubted she would be able to walk again and thought paralysis was a strong possibility.

ARE ANSWERS TO PRAYERS MIRACLES?

A friend of mine who knew of many of the previous successful long-distance healings I had conducted called and asked if I could help Emily, even though Emily was a thousand miles from me. I personally have been through many accidents and much pain and suffering in my seventy-plus years and have always been uplifted and healed, partly because of my strong intent to heal rather than give in to pain or dis-ease. My faith continues to deepen in that which is the Source of all healing energies because of the many healings I have seen and been part of making happen.

After a short time of prayer and reflection to tune in to her conditions, I began assessing Emily's body. As I have mentioned (but it bears repeating), space and time present no barriers to energy medicine, healing energy, or prayer, or to our perception, if we develop it fully. I saw with my inner eye a huge disruption in the bioelectric energy field around Emily's body and began to work energetically to bring it into balance so it could help stabilize her body and bring her into coherence.

Once I sensed there was more stability, I again scanned Emily's body. I noted that her spinal canal had been narrowed (a condition called *stenosis*) in the cervical (neck) area, which nonetheless appeared to be intact and not seriously injured. I was certain then that she would not be paralyzed.

Next I examined the cervical disks and vertebrae and saw some damage. I used healing intention and focusing skills—which anyone can learn to use, with practice—to bring the cervical spine area to a state where it would repair more quickly. As I do this scanning with my clients, I actually see new cells forming—trillions of them coming from the light in and around the client. You might say this is the original blueprint of health for each one of us. As the new cells come in, the old, damaged ones are cast off by the body through the circulatory and other elimination systems, such as the breath.

As I do with many of my critically ill or injured clients, I maintained my awareness of Emily during the days that followed, sending healing energies to the injured areas. When I consciously merged my perceptions with her from time to time, I could see that her body was very gradually accepting the healing energies, building new cells to replace the damaged ones at a faster rate than they had at first.

To be a positive healer or to have positive prayer, we must place no conditions on what occurs other than our intention to do the best that we can. It is important to know that guidance is ever-present, just as when we might intuitively pray for a loved one and find out later that person was in a crisis of some kind at the exact time we felt the desire to pray.

In a week, Emily was able to leave the hospital for a short stay in a rehabilitation facility and by that time could even take a step or two on her own using a cane. The doctors could not explain her quick recovery, and Emily's family members were calling her recovery "a miracle."

Answers to prayers can be called miracles, but they are not really supernatural at all. They are now and always have been part of the human experience. It is a natural process—the law of attraction, if you will—that supplies answers when we sincerely ask for help. Healing intent incorporates positive expectation of well-being through deep, sustained focus. This is what I do when I see my clients as being energetically present with me. It allows for a healing to occur. Positive intentions raise the frequency of the body and, together with the desire of a client to accept healing, allow healing energies to integrate into the client wherever there is need for healing—mentally, emotionally, spiritually, and physically.

INTENT TO HEAL OVER DISTANCES AND THERAPEUTIC TOUCH

Dolores Krieger and Dora van Gelder Kunz started the therapeutic touch movement for medical and other health professionals more than thirty years ago. Today thousands of nurses, medical doctors, and other health providers worldwide use the principles of therapeutic touch to help patients heal from both minor difficulties and major illnesses, including cancer.

One of the attributes of therapeutic touch is that the practitioners are trained to develop intention to help heal. Another is that physical touching is not necessary to transfer healing energy; instead, being centered, peaceful, and focused with one's intent is of paramount importance. Researchers have studied the effects of therapeutic touch for the last thirty years, coining the acronym NCTT (non-contact therapeutic touch). Placebo-controlled studies have shown that NCTT helps wounds heal faster than a placebo, lowers blood pressure, and, at least anecdotally, helps heal severe illnesses and dis-eases.

SARAH'S BREATHING IMPROVES WITH LONG-DISTANCE HEALING

Distance, no matter how great, is not a barrier to the transfer of focused healing energy. The healer simply intends to be a channel for healing energy from universal Source to the patient. Consciousness delivers. There are many examples of positive outcomes from long-distance healing in just my work alone, including the case of Sarah Jones, now almost 80. Sarah had been a friend of mine for several years; eventually she became a regular client. She called for help because, for some time, she had not been able to breathe deeply. She noticed the condition getting rapidly worse. Her main concern was her lung capacity. She also had a secondary difficulty in that she could not breathe through her nose at all. She attributed the latter to chronic sinus congestion.

Sarah called me because she knew of my medical intuitive work and the energy healings I had conducted for many other people. She said she wanted me to work with her because she knew she was in trouble. I could tell she had a deep commitment to her healing and the confidence that it could be achieved.

During our first telephone session, I found out that Sarah had been a smoker for more than thirty years and had stopped smoking ten years earlier. I sensed that her healing was going to be a challenge, and as our regular appointments progressed, my hunch turned out to be correct. I knew that she breathed with the assistance of an oxygen concentrator at night. She also sometimes used it during the day, as she would become breathless after even slight exertion.

Sarah asked me to work on opening her sinuses before moving to her lungs, as she was completely unable to breathe through her nose. I began using healing energies to help clear her nasal passages and sinuses. As I sat in my office two thousand miles away from Sarah, with my telephone earpiece on, I held my hands out as if she was sitting just in front of me and began to focus my intent.

I put my hands up to the area where her sinuses would be if she had been sitting before me and began focusing healing energy there. I could feel the energy flowing through my hands to the area of Sarah's sinus cavities, and she reported that she was beginning to experience some relief there. She knew I had intuitive sight, so at this point she asked if I would look into her lungs. When I did, I could see the cilia and damaged alveoli pockets, and I knew we had a major challenge. I told Sarah it might take several sessions for us to accomplish her healing together, and she said she was ready.

Our next task was to begin relaxing the musculature involved with Sarah's rib cage, as it needed to be more flexible in order for her lungs to expand and contract more fully. The whole area was quite stiff in the beginning, and as I channeled the healing energy—and Sarah assisted by being aligned with the work and allowing the healing—she began to experience a sense of the energy working within her body. She soon could feel a greater sense of relaxation and flexibility in her rib cage.

I then focused on her lungs, and soon she reported that she was beginning to breathe more easily. Each time we worked together, her breathing capacity grew. I could see the healing in her lungs. Sometimes Sarah would ask me how the cilia looked, and each time I could say that they looked improved from the time before. Cilia are slender, brush-like protuberances that line the lungs and sweep fluids and toxins out. I saw the cilia as being stronger and moving more easily in the respiration process.

Each time we worked together energetically, I would ask Sarah if she was still feeling improvement, and she always affirmed feeling increasingly better. I could see that the damage in her alveoli pockets was healing. However, in one of our last sessions together, she remarked that she had gotten tired and was not sure whether she was continuing to improve. When we had started working together four months earlier, Sarah could only take a few steps before she had to sit down and breathe straight oxygen to get her breath back. I asked her what improvement she had noticed since that time, and she said that there was no comparison because she felt so much better. I asked her why she wondered whether she was continuing to improve, and she said, "Well, my daughter-in-law and I planted six 50-foot rows of squash, peppers, and a little bit of this and that today, and I got tired." I could not even imagine myself at age eighty doing what she had just done in her garden!

Sarah called some weeks later and said she had planted ten more rows of vegetables and picked the first squashes and peppers from her original plantings. She also mentioned that she had seen her doctor recently—and he confirmed that she was breathing much better, although he could not explain why.

20

Hepatitis C, Energy Medicine, and Turning a Challenge into a Success Story

> ***Everyone knows what they want; they just dismiss it because they don't believe they can have it.***
>
> **—TREVOR CAMPBELL, in *The Magician's Way***

At least once each day I take the opportunity to sit down and spend peaceful moments reflecting on my clients. So very many of them have turned their health challenges into success stories. These are courageous people who have been steadfast in their commitments to achieve health in body, mind, and spirit through very difficult circumstances.

Ted is one such example. He called me and asked if I had ever had success helping someone reverse hepatitis C using energy medicine. I remembered working with several people who had hepatitis C. Each one had improved after treatments with energy medicine and the implementation of a healthy diet and lifestyle changes.

I discussed with Ted the fact that hepatitis C is a viral infection accompanied by inflammation of the liver; this, in some people, can lead to cirrhosis and even the need for a liver transplant—and, in severe cases, death. He told me that he had been infected through a blood transfusion. Hepatitis C can only be passed from human to human by blood transmission of some kind. Because he had not yet experienced fibrosis—scarring of the liver—Ted thought there could be a chance of remission or healing.

Hepatitis C has a reputation of being very serious, even though only one-third of patients with the chronic type develop cirrhosis within twenty years. Other issues that may arise are fatigue, flu-like symptoms, joint pains, itching, sleep disturbances, appetite changes, nausea, and depression. Ted had no time to lose in his healing process, as he had experienced several of these symptoms and was losing weight.

HEALING WITH LIGHT FROM THE ORIGINAL BLUEPRINT

Ted agreed to meet by phone every two weeks for energy healing. For me, this process involves pulling pure light from the centers of healthy cells—actually, from the original blueprint of the cells—and with focused intent, orchestrating the replacement of the unhealthy cells with cells possessing the original healthy cell structure.

Ted and I also discussed the lifestyle and dietary changes he had already made and those he might need to make. In one of our early meetings he disclosed that he had not truly committed to the challenge ahead. For example, although he wanted to heal his condition, he had eaten unhealthy lunches with "the boys" several times after we had begun our work together, and he had paid for it with liver pain that sometimes lasted for three or four days. Each time this happened, we had to start over again with the cellular healing.

Almost everyone has the ability to stay focused, and it is important to do so in any healing endeavor. In my practice, because of the medical intuition I was born with, clients cannot slip one past me. I know whether someone has a true commitment to health; when they are committed, the healing will begin to manifest and be recognized by the body starting with the cells, which connect to the original source of their light.

THE IMPORTANCE OF MAKING A COMPLETE COMMITMENT

I could only truly begin the work of helping heal Ted's liver when he made a complete commitment to that work. Such is the case with all healing; the person desiring the healing must be committed to changing whatever needs to be changed in order for the health he or she desires to manifest. If there is the slightest sense of wanting to hold on to a condition, to keep things the same, it will prevent healing. We talked of this, and Ted eventually agreed that he would honor the process of fully healing his liver no matter what it would take.

I explained my intent to bring forward trillions of new, healthy cells from deep within the light of his physical body, as well as from energy fields around his body, to replace the damaged cells. I can spiritually see both the unhealthy cells and the new, healthy ones. I can also help the body to flush out the damaged cells, such as those in Ted's liver. His liver was unable to do the work itself because of the dis-ease. It is important to note again that I can only help in this way if someone is completely and unequivocally committed to healing.

THE LIGHT OF THE CELLS

This light of the cells, which I can clearly see, may be recognized by many readers as the light that has been scientifically proven by physicists to be the basis of our physical bodies. The world-renowned physicist David Bohm speaks of matter as slowed-down light. He says, "Light is what enfolds the universe. In its generalized sense, it is the means by which the entire universe unfolds into itself. It is energy, information, content, form and structure. It is the potential of everything."[1]

I have learned, through many years of energy healing experiences, how to focus my consciousness and go to the center of new cells—cells the body creates all the time, but that can be encouraged to grow faster by healing intent. I see where the light of life resides in each of these cells, and I work with my clients to bring this original light through in a stronger way so that a new, healthy cell will replace the old, damaged one.

THE INTELLIGENCE OF CELLS

Remarkably, the new cells seem to know exactly where to grow. It is as if they are guided by a great Source intelligence. The sick cells are unable to sustain health, and thus they are released by the regular eliminatory methods of the body.

Ted's awareness was a very important factor in the healing work we did together. I learned that he could accurately feel the energies swirling in and around his liver as we focused our intent. He was able to sense each step of the process, from the moment I began to scan his liver through the time when I saw trillions of light cells forming and swept the old ones away. Ted told me he could tell when changes were taking place; when my invisible, energetic hands were layering new cells; and when I stopped.

Actually, anyone can do healing like this with the right intent and focus. It just takes practice, and since I have been doing it for most of my life, it seems to come naturally. Still, I cannot do healing work for anyone who is not honestly 100 percent committed to the process of their own healing. Cells of the body are that intelligent. They follow thought.

I have been a clinical nutritionist for many years, and I almost always focus on the nutritional aspects of healing with my clients. Although I cannot prescribe medicines, I can tell them what I would take if I were in their shoes. During our sessions, Ted and I discussed the importance of taking nutritional supplements that would support his liver, such as milk thistle extract. I learned that Ted had been on a health-conscious path for a few years, and it was only when he began to feel quite ill from the hepatitis C that he fell away from his commitment to health and wellness.

Only several months later, when he felt much stronger, did Ted tell me that prior to the beginning of our work together, he had lost more than twenty-five pounds—a loss that he could ill afford. By the time our healing sessions were over, he had regained all the weight. During the course of my energetic assistance, Ted's faith in his own healing journey and his commitment to lifestyle and dietary changes were vital to his healing. Such a commitment can make a difference between a very poor quality of life and a very good one.

21

Healing Emotional Conditions

The first time you experience unconditional love as an adult, it may be a gentle melting of a glacier. Or it may be more of a cataclysm, like a giant earthquake that shakes you to your inner core. You are falling in love, but the act of receiving love that intense and all encompassing changes your conception of yourself. You can't swim in such a vast ocean and remain entirely in the small pond of your limited self. Even if that opening is only for an instant, even if it goes away and is apparently forgotten, that moment of realization, of the heart opening, colors the rest of a lifetime.

—RAM DASS, *Be Love Now*

Once in a while, a client requests a physical healing that involves much more than just the physical body. As an intuitive healer, I am acutely aware that deeper levels of healing may also need to take place in order for a person to be healed physically. Trish came to me for healing an inability to breathe deeply, which she said was caused by old illnesses. She said her lungs were beginning to stiffen, but it was clear to me that she was being affected by emotional issues involving members of her family. Initially, however, Trish did not realize how her journey toward physical healing would first lead us into her emotional healing.

LETTING GO CREATES SHIFTS IN THE BODY

One of the basic principles of the healing work I do, as I have said—but it bears repeating since it is so important—is that the client must make a commitment that true healing is what he or she desires; usually, first I know whether the client has made this commitment either consciously or energetically, and then I elicit a verbal commitment during the course of our conversation. When the client is ready to let go of the dis-ease, and when I feel the release of the negative energies associated with that condition, I can "see" internal shifts taking place in the body, allowing purer and lighter energies to replace the old everywhere in the body and energetic field.

Trish's intent was strong and pure, and her focus clearly was on healing "whatever it takes to become whole"; her trust in me as an ally to help her heal was also strong, and so we began. At first we worked with her childhood abuses, as they had been affecting her adult life in ways that strangled her relationship with her husband. As I worked with her, I sensed how other family members had become a part of her story and how she perceived them negatively, thus detrimentally affecting her health. Healing had to take place, and I suggested several Emotional Freedom Technique (EFT) sessions to facilitate the release of detrimental thoughts and energies in order to assist the healing process. This process was vital for her so that she could free herself from past perceptions and experiences that were affecting her in the present.

We addressed the need for a commitment on Trish's part to self-forgive—a commitment not only to make the time to practice forgiveness in order to release any judgments against herself and any other people involved, but also to marshal the focus and intent necessary to forgive herself at very deep levels. She practiced until she could feel the healing of deep self-love. Then she was able to take the EFT steps toward her own personal freedom by choosing statements that helped her release negative emotions. Throughout this process, I held a vision of her being whole, and I could sense shifts taking place as she let go of past traumas and judgments.

Together we built a new foundation upon which Trish could easily stand. She became aware of the possibilities of new and healthy connections with her family and other loved ones. Her release of the negative also brought her a step closer to physical healing. She began to trust her own intuition, and the transition from me being the intuitive healer gradually shifted over to this woman embracing her ability to allow healing for herself. Self-respect, courage, singular intent, and focus were essential to her healing.

ARE YOU READY?

I always ask each client the question, "Are you ready?" Their answers allow me to see what emotional or thought issues must be dealt with first in the event that they are not fully ready (even if they verbally say yes). Then, after we work through the issues that are blocking a full "yes," I am gratified to hear a solid, 100 percent committed "yes." Through the experiences I have had with many people over many years, a pattern has emerged. It shows me that there may be reservations at first, but if the person is sincere, healing will take place.

As a result of her healing, Trish could walk for more than one block without becoming winded, was able to speak to family members without stuttering and gasping for air, and no longer feared criticism from them.

My experiences have shown me that individual healings ripple out to beneficially affect the individual's family—and the larger community. As scientists are now validating through recent discoveries in physics and cell communication, there is no separation other than the belief of separation. It can thus be understood that the healing "ripple effect" continues on forever, as we are all connected on many different levels.

22

The Importance of Alignment with Healing

> ***I understood that I owed it to myself, to everyone I met, and to life itself to always be an expression of my own unique essence. . . . My healing wasn't so much born from a shift in my state of mind or beliefs as it was from finally allowing my true spirit to shine through.***
>
> —**ANITA MOORJANI,** ***Dying to Be Me***

Often, an experience I have with a client leaves me feeling deep gratitude for my education in psychology, nutrition, energy healing, and related subjects. Knowledge in these areas has proven to be an integral part of my practice of intuitive medicine.

For example, I received a call from Florence, a woman who had been diagnosed with breast cancer. After she had done some research, Florence called me to ask if I would be a part of her healing process. She is married to a medical doctor, and she had told him that she was adamant about not going the route of "regular medicine."

Those who call me for help have heard of intuitive medical practitioners, and they fully expect us to be able to view the health of their bodies intuitively over the telephone. In my case, I sometimes perceive the body in its entirety, seeing a whole picture all at once. More often, though, I scan the body from head to toe in a more analytical way. The intuitional capabilities that transcend the five senses are innate in everyone, but in most cases, these are educated out of us at an early age. This was not so in my case, as you now know.

When I assessed Florence's body, I found what appeared to be a small tumor in her breast; I could not tell whether it was benign or cancerous. We discussed her alternatives; she was opposed to any more biopsies. She had already started a program of nutritional supplements that she had found through her own research. In case she wanted to try something different from or in addition to what she was already taking, I suggested other supplements that might be more beneficial during the time of healing.

CANCER AND HABITUAL PATTERNS

Most people who have been diagnosed with cancer have habitual patterns of fear or stressful thoughts. I could tell by the sound of Florence's voice that she was highly stressed. I know when stress is a long-standing pattern in people's lives, and I see it as a precursor to dis-eases that might later be diagnosed by a physician. Florence disclosed her emotional difficulties, fears, and challenges, and I recommended EFT, which she could use to reduce her stress and thereby help the healing of any cancer.

Florence continued our telephone consultations for the next several weeks and made adjustments to her nutrition and supplements. During her first appointment, I had started sending her non-contact healing energy, a technique I discussed earlier, and one that many doctors and nurses now use and anyone can learn to do. I do this with my clients until there is a healing, and I direct this positive healing energy according to the perceptions I receive about their challenges.

ONE HUNDRED PERCENT ALIGNMENT WITH HEALING

After four sessions, I ascertained that Florence was fully healed when I scanned her body and no longer perceived the small tumor I had previously intuitively seen. She also felt that her breast was free of what could have been a cancerous tumor. A subsequent mammogram showed no tumor or mass, and she was declared clear. This healing happened because Florence was 100 percent aligned with healing, and she allowed the healing energy that I channeled to work within her. This energy, her commitment, and the nutritional supplements all combined to effect the healing.

When Florence told her physician husband, he was pleased that she was healed but was surprised at how it had happened. Between our phone sessions, she had followed my suggestions to do emotional release practices, such as practicing forgiveness for anything within herself that she had been judging or criticizing. I could feel the positive difference during each ensuing session. I noticed that her voice was calmer and she was more direct in her words as she described successes in her release work.

The art of allowing, of accepting self and others without making judgments, is also important for the healer to be fully aligned with healing. We are all fundamentally involved in creating our own health, and being focused on health for each person we meet helps draw it out and to ourselves, as well.

23

Resolving Conflicting Beliefs

I cast my own shadow upon my path, because I have a lamp that has not been lighted.

—RABINDRANATH TAGORE, *"Stray Birds" CIX*

Oprah Winfrey, on one of her widely watched daytime television shows, made the statement that we are all energetic beings, meaning we are all made up of energy. She was talking with Mehmet Oz, who was a regular guest on her show at the time and who had been describing to Oprah's audience the energetic workings of the human body and energy fields around the body.

INVISIBLE FORCES IN OUR BODIES

It is true that our bodies are made of energy and that they are influenced by perhaps thousands of subtle energy fields and other currents that flow through and around them. These fields could be described as invisible forces that move in and out of all living things. One example is the energy from the sun, which affects plants, trees, and literally every body on the earth; in fact, scientists are now postulating that even our sun is powered by galactic electric currents that converge on it, making its light more like lightning than a product of nuclear fusion.[1] Too, our own powerful feelings and thoughts are energies. All of these affect our health.

I think it is useful to understand how healing takes place primarily on energetic levels. Healing of the physical so often comes from unseen energies directed by thought and desire. Neurological impulses are often stimulated when our bodies receive an energetic impact from someone or something, such as a burst of anger from someone close or a feeling of deep love one has toward another. Because our bodies are not only energetically but also electrically based, they, too, can influence our feelings; for example, we tend to feel happy when it is sunny as well as when someone smiles at us. The sunshine stimulates hormones, and the smile does, too.

It bears repeating that our thoughts also have power and energy; they immediately affect our DNA and thus cellular function throughout the body. We have all had the feeling of wanting to move ourselves away from someone who is talking about negative things—we may say we do not want to be "caught up in that negativity." And when we are with people who are happy and laughing, we are attracted to them and want to spend time with them. Thoughts are like magnets, either attracting or repelling. It is therefore important to be aware of thoughts and feelings at all times.

THE EFFECT OF ENGAGING WITH DISRUPTIVE ENERGIES AROUND US

Often we can sense others' thoughts, even if only at a subconscious level. Some of us are more sensitive to the subtle energy of thoughts than others, but we all are potentially affected in some way. This energy can significantly affect our health, which is something I often address in my work as a medical intuitive. In addition to the energy of negativity itself and how it can cause harm, new research shows that negative feelings underlying our hurt feelings can cause heart failure if the feelings are unresolved. Our beliefs about past events can create cardiovascular disease through tension, inflammation, and high blood pressure.[2]

Frequently when I am helping a client, I suggest that the person can become healed of physical illnesses often associated with negative thinking by changing his or her thoughts to a more positive energy. Napoleon Hill, in his famous book *Think and Grow Rich*, wrote that a person becomes what he thinks about all day long. It is easy to realize the truth that thought produces effects when we look around at the manifestations of thought in the lives of people we know and work with, and even ourselves. You can see how a negative thought about someone will cause you to be judgmental about that person, but judgment always creates tension. I know that the notion that we create much of what occurs in our own lives is controversial, yet I see it play out all the time.

A CASE SHOWING HOW THOUGHTS AFFECT THE BODY

Janice had been worrying for years about a recurrence of a cancer that had been present in her body due to an energetic imbalance. She was very anxious when she called and asked me to scan her body and then tell her what I saw energetically. According to a recent blood test, Janice had markers for cancer, and the doctors had told her that an illness must be hiding in her body. I told her that I saw her as being healthy at that moment. I did not see any pockets where the cancer was supposed to be hiding. She pointed out that I had told her the same thing—that she was healthy—six months earlier, and other energetic healers she had called had also told her that she was basically healthy, yet the medical community told her she was getting sicker, although they could not find out why. Nothing showed up other than the negative markers in her blood tests.

I find this case interesting with respect to how thoughts influence the physical body. Earlier in my life, as part of my degree program at the University of California, Los Angeles, I did an experiment to see if I could influence the results of my own blood tests with my thoughts. The first blood test was performed after I deliberately focused on an emotionally negative experience I had when I was younger. The blood drawn during this negative focus showed clumping blood cells and anemia. That same day, in the same lab, I took a second test, but before I did, I listened to some of my favorite music (Mozart and Chopin) and looked at photos of happy faces and at pictures of places I had experienced with joy. When I felt my thoughts and emotions shift to the positive, I had more blood drawn. When it was analyzed, the blood was very healthy, with no clumping cells, and it was no longer anemic.

I knew from that experience that thoughts influence outcomes. What was happening with Janice was that she had not been challenging herself to focus on anything positive, not even what she had been told by the healers she had called. She was clinging to the results of blood tests that made her believe her body was crumbling. I began to wonder if it was her negative expectation, a *nocebo*, that had influenced the blood tests.

Janice and I talked about her confusing beliefs. She had sought advice from alternative sources but chose not to put credence in what they said. She had a preconceived belief that the blood tests were more accurate than what she was hearing from her alternative health practitioners. We also discussed her fear of being judged if she did succumb to the cancer she was afraid was eating away at her body. Then we talked of how she could change her thoughts by accepting only those suggestions that supported health. This would be a huge step for her, as she had always listened to others' advice, and after seeking out so many opinions, she no longer knew what to believe.

Janice's energy fields were muddled and looked as if they, too, were taking instructions from a myriad of sources. I suggested that Janice take a vacation from all the people who were negating any positive outcome and begin clearing any negative beliefs that she knew did not serve her desire for health. I also suggested she begin focusing on the positive input she was receiving from medical intuitives, body workers, holistic nutritionists, and others she had been seeing. The negativity that plagued her mind could be banished by consciously monitoring her thoughts and choosing those that were aligned with health, peace, happiness, and a deep sense of well-being.

Most of my clients have used illness as a way to get attention from someone else. This was true of Janice as well, and I suggested to her that she might consider whether she was using illness to get attention. When this is the case, it gives someone a reason to keep themselves ill. She called me one week later and told me I was right. She said that after the session, when she realized she had been using illness as a way to get attention for herself, she cried for an hour.

It is absolutely essential that a person requesting a healing of body, mind, and spirit must find some place to retreat, whether it is a healing center or a peaceful room in the midst of daily life, where he or she can be quiet and rest for a time; pull forward positive energy, positive thoughts, and positive feelings; and bring peace, quiet, reflection, and healing by desire and intention. Most of us have the ability to energetically create a healing place wherever we are and to surrender to the healing energies we request. Sometimes lighting a candle, reading a poem, gazing upon a flower, or listening to peaceful music can set the stage for an energetic transformation to health. Some people are too weak or sick to create their own healing space, so it is important to be sensitive to the needs of others and help them find what will bring them a sense of peace as they begin their healing.

24

Obsessive-Compulsive Behavior and How Feeling Good Enough Opens the Doors to Healing

> ***If things go wrong in the world, this is because something is wrong with the individual, because something is wrong with me. Therefore, if I am sensible, I shall put myself right first.***
>
> **—CARL JUNG, in *The Collected Works of C. G. Jung***

Sophie, a woman in her late thirties, first telephoned me to ask about a chemical imbalance (allergies) in her body. I felt it was important to start slowly with her, as I could sense that she was in a delicate emotional state. I knew intuitively that there was trauma stored in her energy field, and I could see it had started at the time her son was born. I could also see that there were unresolved emotions from events in her own childhood. I thought addressing both of these issues was central to her healing.

THE BENEFITS OF EXERCISE, ENDORPHINS, AND OXYGEN

I suggested that Sophie start an exercise routine to get her endorphins flowing and provide more oxygen to her body. What I knew was that the endorphins and oxygen would move her into not only a state of receptivity, but also a feeling of more health and well-being flowing to her. After this discussion during the first part of our phone call, she asked me if I would be willing to use my intuitive insights about her to help resolve some difficult emotions and also coach her about nutrition for her family.

ANXIETY AND REPETITIVE THOUGHTS

Sophie disclosed that she kept thinking the same things over and over and doing things over and over, such as rearranging her kitchen cupboards, thinking she could not get it quite right. She said she thought she was overly critical and too fastidious in some ways. I asked her if she knew anything about people who are obsessive-compulsive. She paused and then said, "You know, sometimes I wonder if I have that." Then, because she wanted to know, a door opened inside her, and I knew at that point I would be able to help her.

Sophie said she had a deep fear that she could be suffering from obsessive-compulsive disorder. She was also afraid that her children could inherit this disorder from her, as one of her young children had exhibited what she feared was the same thing. I did not want to say more at this point regarding what I intuitively sensed about her first child. I wanted to guide her to the point where she would have her own insights and then talk about them.

Using energy medicine techniques, I began to smooth the sharp sparks of energy that I saw charging out of her energy field from her anxiety. At that point, I also suggested she begin keeping a journal. In her next phone call, Sophie told me she had started writing in the journal. In the process, she regained the memory of herself as a very young girl standing in front of an immense door at her great-aunt's home, so paralyzed with dread and fear that she could not bear to go through that door. She had a fear of the smells in the home and the way her great-aunt would treat her. She never felt good enough in her great-aunt's eyes.

THE ROOTS OF OBSESSIVE THOUGHTS

Sophie and I worked together to uncover the origins of this disorder, which had started in early childhood. Her parents had constantly questioned her about what she was doing in school and why her hair was not combed correctly. She said she had compulsively complained to her father about things that bothered her, but in turn, he criticized her for complaining. If he asked her how she was, instead of saying "just fine," she would be honest and tell her father how she felt. She never felt that she was good enough, and when she told him her feelings, it just reinforced this issue because he criticized her. This vicious cycle with her father had never been resolved for Sophie.

Once this memory surfaced, I felt we could start the process of healing. If Sophie could shift her dread and fear, it would contribute to a much healthier approach to life for her.

There was an additional factor compounding these issues: the dread was from her childhood, but the fear was more related to memories of 9/11 and the twin towers. One of her children was born in New York City a day after the twin towers were destroyed. Three of her husband's friends died in the towers, and she felt abandoned by him as he searched for them and grieved that loss instead of staying with her while she was in labor with their child.

Sophie knew I had been using energy medicine with her while we talked; she said she could feel the energy moving and that she felt calmer. She could feel me pulling negative emotional energy out of her field and replacing it with feelings of unconditional love. I encouraged her to take time each day to forgive herself for any negative thoughts and feelings she had—toward herself first, and then toward others. She reacted positively and later told me she was doing this practice every day.

TRACKING OBSESSIVE THOUGHTS AND BEHAVIORS

At my suggestion, Sophie had begun tracking her behaviors by noting them in her journal. She made a list of those obsessive-compulsive thoughts and actions she caught herself doing. Each time we talked, we addressed these things and how they played out in her life. Once she saw the pattern, I suggested she stop whatever habit she was performing in mid-step or mid-thought; in other words, she could consciously break the habit and replace it with feelings of harmony in her life.

Sophie is very committed to her self-healing as well as the mental, emotional, and physical health of her children. She diligently practiced self-awareness, catching herself in compulsive or obsessive thoughts and behaviors and making notes when she had insights. These notes would help her become aware of similar patterns in her children. Each time we talked, I sensed more peace and stability within her, and her voice became lighter, her energies brighter. Within two months, Sophie had begun to create new ways of outwardly expressing the inner peace she finally felt.

25

Resilience and Forgiveness

Keys to Health

Healing may not be so much about getting better, as about letting go of everything that isn't you—all of the expectations, all of the beliefs—and becoming who you are.

—RACHEL NAOMI REMEN, in *Healing and the Mind*

We are basically beings who know that we are worthy and that life is supposed to feel good to us. Anything contrary is just a belief we have either inherited or formed. When things do not feel easy, it is because we are resisting the natural flow of life due to some thought or belief.

KEYS TO HEALTH: A CASE HISTORY

Many times over the years, as I have listened to my clients' stories of pain and other challenges, I have been amazed and heartened by their resilience. Resilience is all around us. Merriam-Webster's online dictionary defines the word *resilience* as "an ability to recover from or adjust easily to misfortune or change." A close friend of mine has described it as "to keep on keeping on, in spite of appearances all around you."

Very brave individuals can and do teach the rest of us how to live in the moment, how to face extra physical challenges with courage, and how to make choices that many of us instinctively cringe and run away from making. Life becomes more precious as we realize how to live in the present when faced with a challenge; being in the moment, not looking backward or forward too much, has a presence and power about it.

In his book *The Power of Now,* Eckhart Tolle writes about surrendering or yielding to—rather than fighting—the flow of life, in all its seen and unseen presence. Tolle writes, "Surrender is to accept the present moment unconditionally and without reservation."[1] This quality seems to be the core of healing in many of my clients. As we begin our healing work together, they surrender to a greater power of life and become more resilient to their circumstances; they adjust easily to living in the now, in each moment, as it happens.

MAKING SURE CANCER DOES NOT RETURN

Kathryn is a delightful woman who called me for help. She had already experienced cancer in her lungs, breasts, and part of her spine and had finished as much chemotherapy treatment as the oncologists would permit. She had had radiation treatments, as well. She began to look for alternative treatments and consulted with a few medical intuitives. She decided to work with me to rebuild her health.

Kathryn had learned about the importance of positive thinking and focusing on what she wanted—a totally healthy body. However, as she was now in remission, she wanted to work with me to make sure no cancers returned. We had infrequent appointments, usually two months apart; she scheduled them to occur just before she was to have blood tests that would show what her cancer markers were. We conducted our appointments over the phone immediately before the tests so that she would be as mentally positive as possible.

Kathryn would ask me to intuitively scan her body. After scanning, I would tell her what I saw, and each time she seemed to me to be cancer-free. The test markers confirmed that she was holding her own. However, I realized early on that she was obsessing about the blood tests and their results and was quite fearful that the markers might change. I strongly urged her to evaluate how she was thinking and feeling. I knew that she needed to adjust her attitude if she wanted to remain healthy and that we needed to work together to give her something positive to focus on instead of her fear, which was actually energizing what she did not want. I told her that what you fear, you draw to you, and what you focus on comes to you, as well.

I emphasized that it would benefit Kathryn to become more positive about the fact that she was already in remission and to accept health rather than dwell on past fears. She had started withdrawing from friends and former co-workers when she was diagnosed with cancer, so I suggested that she start reaching out to these people whom she had shut out of her small support group, and also to begin walking with neighbors whom she had walked with before. She agreed.

I gave Kathryn the assignment to practice as completely as she could a very simple exercise, one that I frequently give to my clients to help them bring forward positive healing energy. The focus of this exercise is to forgive oneself for any negative thoughts, judgments, and memories about others. After that has been accomplished, one can begin forgiving the circumstances, experiences, and other people involved.

I have found that people may attempt to forgive others, but they undoubtedly will continue to judge those others unless they first forgive themselves. Healing truly occurs only when you forgive yourself. I knew that this was important for Kathryn in her work. She had had painful, abusive experiences with her stepfather. These painful experiences had helped create an unhealthy pattern that affected her ability to be vulnerable with others, and she had shut part of herself down.

After that phone call was over, I did not know if Kathryn would make any further appointments with me, as I had been very firm with her in regard to the need for her to shift her focus toward the positive outcome she wanted. Two months later, Kathryn called for another appointment. She had some exciting news. She had done her forgiveness work. She had stopped worrying about her blood tests, and her latest test results had turned out to be better than expected. Her most exciting news was that she and her husband had been able to begin talking about what it would be like to live in the present moment. He told her he had been waiting for so long to hear her say she was ready to accept each day as fresh and new, and focus on being healthy.

Not only did Kathryn stay in remission, but she gained so much more than she had ever imagined by exchanging the emotions of fear and dread with a fresh outlook on life. With her husband at her side, she began to plan a cruise around the world as well as other adventures that, in her past, had seemed impossible. Kathryn learned how to become resilient and surrender to the now, living each moment in peace and health. All it took was self-forgiveness and a focus on what she wanted: health, which is here, powerfully, for all of us, in the ever-present now.

26

A Case of Sinus Pain and Infections

Unless you are in a state of alignment with the love that Source flows to you, it is as if it is not really there, when, in fact, it is always there.

—JERRY AND ESTHER HICKS, *Getting into the Vortex*

I have worked with many clients to help them heal sinus issues. Sinus pain and congestion often have an emotional component. That is to say, unprocessed emotions—hurt feelings that are unreleased, for example—can cause sinus difficulties. Over time, I noticed that crying sessions often relieved the sinus congestion and pain. Tears contain toxins, whether from environmental factors or repressed emotions, and the release of them through crying or even laughter can be healing.

EMOTIONS, CRYING, AND SINUS RELIEF

The story of one of my cases offers a good example of how crying can release sinus pain and congestion. Patricia had called for help every week for months. She had terrible sinus congestion and had even undergone surgery for the problem. I knew intuitively that she needed to cry, but while it is easy to advise someone to do so, it may be difficult for a person to just start crying.

Patricia was having so many problems in her relationships that she had not had time to process all her emotions. I could hear the nasal tone in her voice, as I was working with her on a regular basis. She eventually disclosed the problems she had with her sinuses. She was carrying several years' worth of emotional baggage that she had not dealt with. Then an interesting thing happened during the healing of her sinuses. She had a car accident, which completely wrecked the car; she loved the car so much that it made her cry to think of what had happened to it. She cried extensively after the accident.

The next time Patricia called, which was just after the car accident and the crying, her sinuses were significantly better. They were so much better that it was apparent to me the crying had helped her release a lot of the emotional energy that had been affecting her sinuses. We then worked together to help her release more of the emotions related to her car accident. At this point I noticed that her sinuses were again significantly improved.

As the months went by, more clients were calling for help with sinus problems than for any other particular condition. Since there were so many clients with sinus challenges, I began looking for patterns in what types of conditions might be causing their symptoms. All of my clients had symptoms related to some or all of the following: geographical region, time of year, food allergies, environment, proximity to animals, mold, weather, and emotions. Many who called wanted sinus pain relief sessions, while others were in the midst of a crisis with sinus inflammation and infection. Most who were suffering sinus pain were almost paralyzed with the effects of their conditions. The long-distance energy medicine I used helped them heal.

PROOF OF VIRTUAL HEALING

Elizabeth called requesting energy healing for her "terrible sinus headache." As I began the session, I did what I normally do: I visualized my fingers around the area on her forehead and the palms of my hands under her eyes so that I could focus the flow of healing energy there. It helps me to channel the flow of healing energy when I visualize my hands actually being on the area, even if the client is on the phone.

Suddenly, I heard a gasp. I asked Elizabeth what had happened, and she replied that she had looked in the mirror while I was working on her and, in the exact areas where I told her I was working, she saw that her skin was bright red. She said it was startling, but it was not so to me. This happens often with clients when I am channeling healing energy. Such confirmation gives them, as it did Elizabeth, stronger belief in the efficacy of energy medicine. Her sinus headache was gone by the time we finished working together over the phone. Our bodies are truly conductors of electromagnetic energies, and if we allow the healing energies to flow to us, including those from another person or from prayer, we heal faster.

SINUS DIFFICULTIES, MEDICATIONS, AND TOXINS

Alison had severe sinus problems. She said she had started seeing halos around things. She asked her doctor about this, and he cautioned her to stop using certain over-the-counter medicines for sinus congestion and sleep because some of those medicines can create a predisposition for glaucoma. So Alison decided to use safe and natural energy medicine. She called me, and we began a series of sessions focusing on healing her eyes and sinuses. The day after one particular session, during which her sinuses had been extremely stopped up, she called and said they had started draining right after the healing session. She had had ongoing infections, but they began to improve and become less frequent during our work together. When Alison discontinued the medications she had been using, her eyes improved, as well.

Intuitive and energy medicine work needs to be very specific. Sometimes I realize that a client with sinus problems has experienced toxins in the workplace—at times this is an intuitive hunch, and other times, it is because they disclose something to me. For example, one client of mine was affected because a new customer of hers wore perfume that my client was sensitive to. Other clients react to such things as fresh indoor paint.

One mother told me her children had frequently been home from school with allergies and colds. Often, this is due to viruses being passed on by other children, but there may be issues having to do with food allergies, diet, or genetic predisposition affecting the sinuses, as well. Eliminating certain foods such as gluten and dairy products, or replacing moisture-compromised carpets, may be important. Cutting out sugar use opens the door for greater health in many instances. Cancers thrive on sugar, allergies seem to crop up with consumption of excess sugar, and sugar can wreak havoc with the immune system.

There are many causes for sinus difficulties, but finding underlying emotional issues is very common as well. An intuitive medicine practitioner can help clients discover things affecting their health that they may not have been aware of. The body is such a remarkable and malleable instrument, and literally any condition can be made better when one allows and embraces healing energy.

27

Boundaries, Allowing, and Complete Health

Complaint is only possible while living in the suburbs of God.

—HAFIZ, in *Mala of the Heart*

Let us discuss a little more the all-encompassing field of well-being—the basis of all life—and its effect on even the subtlest levels of our DNA. Scientific research confirms that we exist in an interconnected field of energy that is always flowing and, as I see it, is bringing us a constant stream of well-being. This source feeds our bodies and, as a basic physical construct, is characterized by light energy, or slowed-down light waves. We receive nourishment at all times from this energy; it feeds the minutest particles of physical matter as well as cells, and therefore large cellular systems such as organs, and thus, all functions of the body. It has rightly been said that we live by more than food alone.

CONNECTION TO PURE WELL-BEING

It is important to have confidence that what we are connected to is pure well-being—and to accept that it is ultimately a mystery. As the brilliant physicist Max Planck said, "Science cannot solve the ultimate mystery of nature. And this is because, in the last analysis, we ourselves are part of nature and, therefore, part of the mystery that we are trying to solve. Music and art are, to an extent, also attempts to solve or at least to express the mystery. But to my mind, the more we progress with either, the more we are brought into harmony with all nature itself."[1]

We are part of nature, and the issue of our boundaries is a fascinating way to look at how we sometimes can cause our own disharmony or ills as well as heal from them. We see boundary issues each day. For example, you keep the volume on your music player at a respectable level for the situation you are in at any given time. This is a boundary issue of noise, and it concerns respecting the physical space as well as the minds and emotions of others. Similarly, you speak gently rather than loudly in conversation to honor others' space. When someone in your life speaks very loudly, you ask if they are seeking attention or trying to control. You might have to set a boundary with them. Often when you are aware of your own responsibility in regard to boundaries, you are more able to draw and communicate your own boundaries about noise or other factors in a compassionate way with others; doing so helps maintain peace of mind and overall health for yourself, and teaches others about you.

MASTERING THOUGHTS

Boundaries around thoughts are also very important. One way I have been able to heal from even very severe illnesses all my life is by mastering my thoughts; also, I have had some devastating accidents, and I have healed from them as well—beyond what the doctors predicted—by staying focused on a healthy outcome and not giving in to any other thought. Many people have done this. The very thought that we are going to be ill causes a resistance to the flow of health; it is akin to setting a boundary against something positive coming in to your life. Your current condition is not the deciding factor in what will be. Let us look, therefore, at the boundaries of psyche.

Because of my hypersensitivity and intuitive abilities, when I was young I had to learn to keep myself from invading or looking into another's mind, emotions, or physical body. My first memory of the need to hold back my perceptions was of my mother clapping her hand over my mouth. I was about six or seven at the time, but by then there had been many incidents where I had innocently said something about someone that was true or came to be true—true, but socially embarrassing to my mother and the other adults around her.

It is second nature for me to be aware of boundaries around me. I still perceive and feel things from others just as I did as a child, but as an adult, I know even more. I have to intentionally keep my sensitivity closed down unless I am asked to use it. I can feel what is going on in people just by looking at them or saying hello socially, and I have to consciously shut that part of my perception down when I sense it happening. I think this is true of everyone to varying degrees, and it is an example of the importance of being aware of one's own feelings, and therefore boundaries, in all situations.

In some cases, I feel something going on in my body just before a new client calls. Soon I learn that his or her issue is just what I felt prior to the call. I might begin to feel a nervous condition or some condition in a particular organ in my body. At other times, a new client calls and ask for a healing session, and after we make an appointment, I start feeling the person's condition. Of course, I clear it in myself so that I will not be affected by that condition and can then be of assistance to that client.

EFFECTS OF SENSITIVE, CONSCIOUS PERCEPTION

We know of the quantum field effect and the interconnectivity of everything at the level of quanta, but the jumps that take place within this field and via consciousness are just beginning to be understood more by scientific observation and measurement. It is very difficult to measure the movements and effects of consciousness; nevertheless, we can sense them, and the more sensitive we are, the more we sense.

One concrete example of how sensitive perception plays a role in my healing work can be seen in the case of a man named Jim, who had a severe bronchial problem. Just after he called to make an appointment, I began to feel his problem—congestion in the bronchial system—in my body. As soon as I realize that I am being affected by a client's difficulties, I can shut it off, clear it out, or put a boundary around me so that I can have the ability to work, to help heal, without taking on the condition.

WOMEN, ABUSE, AND BOUNDARIES

One example of how boundary issues can manifest has to do with women who find themselves in abusive situations or feel obligated to stay in an abusive relationship. Women in these situations have such stress that it affects not only their emotions, but also their bodies. As I do with all women clients who face this issue, I recently urged several women to consult with an attorney as a step toward emotional and physical freedom from an abusive relationship. This gives them practical, empowering knowledge that will ultimately have an effect on their physical health and help them begin to establish healthy boundaries for themselves.

These women usually need to address boundary issues in at least two ways. One, they need to create more boundaries of respect for themselves; they may not be teaching their mate, and probably others in their lives, enough about their boundaries. Thus, they do not get enough respect. They also do not have a space in the home where they are safe. Two, they may need to create a larger boundary for themselves in their own minds. They may have limited themselves to too small a space within their relationship and to conditions that are out of their control. My suggestion that they go to an attorney or counselor gives them something to do to help them create unlimited self-boundaries, whether physical, emotional, or mental.

LIVING YOUR DREAM

You are not living your dream when you do not set boundaries about yourself—what you will or will not do, agree or not agree to. When you are not living your dream, you are resisting it, and that is the same as resisting well-being. Any serious health issue can arise. For example, a new client of mine named Georgia got breast cancer, and the cause of it was from not setting boundaries. She had stopped nurturing herself; she had stopped listening to her own voice about who she was and what she wanted in her life. She put both her husband and her family's desires first; she tried to please them, and she put her own needs aside. The stress led to the illness.

When Georgia put her own needs aside, her life became very stressful. She did not consciously realize this stress at first. In fact, she did not fully understand how putting her needs behind everyone else was affecting her. It was not until we discussed her patterns and her reactions to herself and her family that she could see how her boundaries were too loose; they were allowing too much for others and not enough for her to have the time to care for herself. Some ways to take care of self include taking down time, meditating, listening to music, being outdoors, and looking at nature. By doing these things, you have time to feel and process your thoughts and return to balance.

Judith had elderly parents, both of whom were slipping into dementia; nevertheless, old family dynamics were there that pushed her buttons. She constantly talked about her parents being "a pain in the butt." She called me with chronic and extraordinary low back pain that could not be relieved by surgery. We worked out ways for her to honor her own boundaries regarding her parents, including doing self-forgiveness exercises and specific meditations for general well-being; her low-back pain disappeared once she had released judgments.

BOUNDARIES AND RESPECT OF SELF AND OTHERS

Now we return to Jim, the man I mentioned at the beginning of this chapter who had the bronchial issue. Jim is quite sensitive. He does not, however, know how to protect himself from outside influences. What plays a role in this is that he had a great need to have connections with others. He does not often go inside himself to find peace in silence, nor does he foster self-reliance and self-assurance. Consequently, since he does not respect his own needs for boundaries, he does not respect the boundaries of others; he is just beginning to understand this. Jim does not listen to his own guidance and instead gets entwined in the needs and boundaries of others. This intertwining not only makes him vulnerable to others' thoughts and feelings, but also affects his immune system, because he does not listen to his guidance about what is good or bad for him. So Jim has limited himself to looking outside for guidance rather than relying on his own guidance system.

Another client, Craig, has had a lot of cervical spine issues; nevertheless, he dances twice a week at social events. He likes dancing with one woman in particular, but every time he dances with her, he has pain radiating from a disc to his shoulder. I inquired about her and what he thought of her, and after a while he began to open up. He talked of his feelings about her, his affection for her, and when he finally completely opened up, he said, "Oh, my gosh, my disc just went back into place." Craig had limited himself by keeping himself from feeling and acknowledging his feelings about this woman—until we talked and he opened up. These unexpected, sudden shifts in people are one of the reasons I love what I do: help others sort out the true causes of pain. I see people open themselves to their own health potential.

We all need to continuously be aware of our personal boundaries. We all have varying degrees of sensitivity, but the more sensitive you are, the more you have to be aware of your boundaries. You can make the decision to be more patient with yourself and others. Try not to do too much in any given day so that you can stay present enough to be aware of your feelings. Boundaries are personal, but they are always active in all parts of life; they are there in all interactions with others, including animals, and in your thoughts and feelings as you watch the news. It is important to be aware of when you start to become emotionally attached to something negative, because it can affect your health. Observe your reactions, but do not judge; just be calm, and change to positive thoughts about something.

Boundaries are important in all social interactions. For example, say you are having a discussion with someone. Notice if the other person is becoming emotionally charged. Can you diffuse the charge for yourself in a peaceful way? Are you becoming charged? What do you need to do to stay peaceful? Notice your body, be aware of your heart rate, and be aware of your surroundings, including the bigger picture of everyone in your city or country. You are tuning in to all of you, and from that center, you can practice being more aware of whether another's negative thinking or action is affecting you negatively. Then you can act to change the situation. Being in your center of peace is being in complete health.

Epilogue

Life after Life and Unseen Helpers

> ***Therefore, since we are surrounded by so great a cloud of witnesses . . . let us run with endurance the race that is set before us.***
>
> *—Hebrews 12:1 ESV*

I would like to tell as many open-minded people as possible that I know, without a doubt, that those loved ones who have made the transition we call death are still with us, just in a different way. How do I know? Well, for me, this knowledge came naturally.

Mehmet Oz has twice interviewed Theresa Caputo on his television show. Oz calls Caputo "the Long Island Medium." She was invited to return to his show by popular request and because, as Oz said, "She blew me away." On her return visit, Caputo said that her number one aid to others is to help them overcome their anxiety, and having communications from those loved ones who have crossed over might help immensely. Oz's team announced the show this way: "Could your loved ones on the other side help relieve your anxiety about your health and the future? Tune in today to watch as [Theresa] stuns audience members by communicating with their lost loved ones right on stage."[1] Caputo said that loved ones who have passed away tend to try to give us messages to help us understand things and to relieve our anxieties about them and about ourselves. Caputo said it was not until she began to acknowledge and assess the information she was getting from extrasensory perception that her anxieties quelled. When she began to express to others what she saw in spirit and the information that came with that, she felt better, especially after giving the information to others that unseen loved ones wanted to provide. Caputo said that when she is talking with others, so much information comes to her that she has had to learn to open to it and to express it to help people.

THE RELIEF OF KNOWING WHAT YOU KNOW

Though I do communicate with the deceased loved ones of many of my clients (and others), I have not done my work on stage. Nevertheless, this show is one more piece of evidence to support the fact that millions of people today have opened their minds to communicating with loved ones who have died and to see that life never ends. Oz asked Caputo, "Do you believe that there are spirits on the other side who are trying to get through to us, and that's the sense that we are having, that's the worry we feel sometimes?" Caputo said yes, she does believe that.

I do as well. I know that many people feel loving spirits around them attempt to contact them, but because of their lack of openness, these people instead feel anxiety. I learned a long time ago, just as Caputo did, that if an intuitive impression or someone on the other side came to me to communicate and I did not express it, I would not feel very good. I would feel stressed and become depressed if I did not acknowledge and express. I often had to write my impressions down or meditate, which is what I highly recommend. Here is a little background about how I developed my skills.

As I wrote earlier, when I was about six or seven, I was so ill for so long, in bed by myself for so many weeks, that I had several out-of-body and near-death experiences. I drifted in and out between consciousness in my body and an awareness of being outside my body so many times that I realized then that dying was very easy and there was nothing to fear. In fact, I had to will myself to stay in my body because it would have felt so good to just go. This woke me up to the fact that there is more to us than meets the eye and that we never really die.

NEAR-DEATH EXPERIENCE

The first near-death experience, or NDE, I remember came when I was very sick. I was in bed most of my first-grade school year. The doctors could not figure out why I did not want to eat and why I seemed to have mini-seizures. I remember wanting to have the same energy to play as the other girls, but I easily got very tired and sickly. My mother insisted I spend most of my time in my bed resting and reading books that she brought to keep me occupied.

I vividly remember one night, when I felt very ill, I thought I was going into another mini-seizure, which for me meant fainting followed by vomiting. However, the slowed beating of my heart and the feeling of being lifted in clouds felt wonderful, so I let myself be lifted into what I called "the mist" and saw beautiful, misty-looking people coming to see me. They wrapped me in a loving embrace, which felt so different from the love that I felt from my parents, and so I relished the feeling of being loved and held so gently. I did not recognize any of these misty-looking people, but I just wanted to remain with them. I felt I was in heaven, and the experience taught me never to fear death or slipping away or being out of body "on the other side." I was in that other realm just long enough to remember it, and then it was as if I was let go and had to slide back into my body. I remember that I weakly called for my mother, who was sleeping in her bedroom at the other end of the long hall that separated my room from my parents' room.

I had many experiences of making a transition from being alive in my body to being aware and conscious somewhere outside my body, and these convinced me at a young age that life goes on forever. At this time of my life, I had never heard of anyone having an out-of-body or near-death experience. Today, of course, such things are common knowledge because of the work of Raymond Moody, Ken Ring, and many other researchers.

SEEING THOSE WHO HAVE DIED

As a girl, I not only lived through near-death experiences and the out-of-body awareness that comes with them, but I also had developed intuitive integration in my life, even though it worried my mother. As a part of my intuitive sensitivities, I realized I could see others who had left their bodies. As I described earlier, my first experience in this regard was when I saw my deceased grandmothers, both of whom had died before I was born, appear to me as I looked at their portraits and longed to know them.

While I was still young, I continued to regularly see and interact with others who had made their transition. Then, when I was twelve, my sister was born. We shared a bedroom, and I was no longer alone so much. Along with the need to focus more on having my sister in my room, I began to shut my extrasensory perceptions down a little. They were, however, still with me. I continued to see people who had died whenever I was with someone who talked about their deceased loved ones.

I can give a more specific example here. When I was eighteen, I had a boyfriend who was an ambulance driver. He would tell me about the people he had driven during his shifts. There were many gruesome stories about people who had been in accidents and died. There were no seat belts or car seats in those days. As he would tell me about the people, I would see them. Some were still caught up in the accident, confused, wondering why they could not be in their bodies or what had happened to them or why their bodies looked the way they did. I would try to help them and guide them.

One way to describe how I see what I see is that the person shows up through a kind of haze between my perception and that person. There is no cut-and-dried boundary line around the haze, but it is definitely there. Imagine the light you can see coming from a movie projector. I see the person as though I am seeing through the projector to the screen. The person I am seeing appears as if on the movie screen, but he or she appears in three-dimensional space. Another way to describe it is that the person appears in front of me as a light, smoky film. Usually he or she is about two feet high, right in front of me. Since I have never seen the person before, I describe what I see to my client; I want to make sure the person who is there in front of me is somehow related to the client before I focus more intently on this spirit. I do such things as describe the hair, eye color, and stature, and, if my client indicates that it could be a grandfather, then I ask more questions to see if it is. If so, then I tune in a little more, which lets the person in spirit get closer to me and communicate.

When I was in my early twenties, I had to put many more boundaries on my perceptions in order to stay focused in this reality. For example, several times when I was driving somewhere and saw a traffic accident, I could see the disarray in the scene, of course, which, in and of itself, is distracting to a driver. But I could also see, with extrasensory perception, the people who had been killed. Sometimes I would stop to help at the scene, and those who were now dead would talk with me. They were confused, and I had to let them know that their body was dead and that they just needed to go to the light. This sort of thing was not easy for me, so, to some extent, I had to put blinders on my extra perceptions. I had to learn how to keep my focus in this reality so that I would not pick up everything about everybody around me, unless someone near me needed to know something specific.

THE MOTHER WHO WANTED BLONDE HAIR

Whenever I am talking with someone and the person mentions that a loved one has died, that person immediately shows up to me. He or she usually just stands back a little bit, being polite, unless I invite the person to communicate. In the cases where I am working with a client who wants to have communication with a loved one who has passed into non-physical, I will ask the person who shows up to say something or give me some kind of sign that is familiar to my client so that we know this is the person my client wants to communicate with.

A recent incident is a good example of how interesting these cases can be. Anne called me specifically because she wanted to communicate with her mother, who had died eight months earlier. She was very distraught during the first part of our phone appointment and was sobbing with grief. She missed her mother very much. I wondered what to do because she was crying so much. I saw a woman appear in front of me, but I wanted to make sure she was Anne's mother, so I asked the woman in spirit for a sign to give Anne to indicate her connection. The woman said, "Tell her I'm trying to make my hair blonde." When I said this to Anne, she stopped crying and burst out laughing.

I was happy, of course, that she was laughing, but I asked her why this made her laugh. She replied, "My mother had dark hair, and she was always trying to make it blonde." This comment by the woman in spirit validated for me as well as her daughter that it was Anne's mother in front of me! This was obviously very healing for my client. The session continued with Anne asking a few more questions of her mother, and her mother's answers. I acted as the go-between, of course. One of the things the mother wanted to convey was to tell her granddaughter, in words she would understand, that her grandmother was in heaven and was happy.

WORKING IN HOSPICE WITH THOSE IN TRANSITION

Although I always had these extrasensory perceptions, when I began volunteering for hospice work, I started to regularly use my abilities to help others in a more focused way. During my early twenties and for two decades after, I had to consciously hold back my extrasensory perceptions for various reasons. I married and had children, then I went to college for many years, finally earning a PhD in psychology. I worked in several different full-time professional jobs over the next twenty years. By the time I was forty-six my children were grown, and that is when I entered hospice volunteer work. I worked both in people's homes and in pastoral care, which was where I helped prepare families for the death of their loved one. I also volunteered in a hospice unit in a hospital.

This work gave me more confidence in using my natural abilities to help others. I stopped questioning my own perceptions, which others could not see, because they were now showing up as a regular and practical part of my everyday life. For the next thirteen years I helped innumerable family members prepare to let go of their loved one by saying to the family such things as "I can see that she is getting ready to pass." I could make a general statement like this when I saw the spirit lifting out of the body. No one else saw this, of course, so I would just gently say what I knew, but I could not tell anyone what I was actually seeing. Of course, I worked with the medical staff, the nurses, and when I saw the heartrate or breathing become erratic, I would call a nurse. But I could see the spirit begin to leave. I could see the point where there was no physical life left in the body.

LOVED ONES HELP WITH TRANSITION

Another example of the kinds of experiences I had in hospice work occurred with Fred, who had just taken his last breath; he kept his eyes open during the time I saw his spirit begin passing out of his body. He looked at me, my husband, his wife, and then he looked at us again as we all sat with him. All during that time he had not taken a breath. I kept wondering if he would breathe again, but he did not. Then he looked up at a forty-five-degree angle with a beautiful, bright smile on his face; I looked there to see what he was looking at and saw a beautiful, golden glow out where Fred's eyes were looking. The glow was around a very beloved being standing there, waiting for him. Fred's face started to glow with great beauty. I saw a pure white light and a tunnel form, and this beloved being and Fred's parents were waiting. At this point, I saw his spirit fully leave his body and go up to them through this tunnel at a forty-five-degree angle. This is the angle I have seen with all the patients I have been with who have made their transition; the spirit leaves the body at this forty-five-degree angle.

Another example I had in hospice, which made me realize how much I could see of the subtle worlds, involved a woman who was dying of brain cancer. I took care of April from the time she was still walking, through the time she could not walk anymore, and up until she made her transition. When she stopped walking, about two months before she died, I often sat with her. Just before she died, many times she would look to her left at the blank wall. She would try to talk to someone at the wall, but she could not form words. Others might have thought she was demented, but I could see that April's deceased mother, grandmother, and grandfather were all there talking with her, getting her ready to make her transition.

There are so many more examples I could give of my hospice years, but it would take another book to do so. A lot of the time I just sat with and listened to people. I heard so many remarkable life stories from those who were about to die. They had nothing to hide. Many people had regrets, but others had none. I finished my work in hospice in 1998 in order to concentrate on my private practice.

I want to focus here on just a few of the client cases I have had that involved requests for me to communicate with loved ones who have crossed over. Often now my clients ask for my help in communicating with their deceased loved ones once they learn I can do this. The visualizing I do when I work with my clients over the phone, as

I have described in previous chapters, seems to stimulate this ability to see those who are alive in spiritual energy.

A SWEET PEA GRANDMOTHER

This case involved a client named Joan, who was having difficulty in many aspects of her life. Toward the end of our first telephone session together, all of a sudden a woman appeared in front of me in spirit. I had a hunch she was Joan's grandmother. Before going further with this story, it may be useful to explain how the appearance of someone who has died, such as Joan's grandmother, occurs for me.

Often, when I am talking with someone about a loved one who has passed away, that person will appear in front of me in an energy form (as I mentioned previously), almost as though I were wearing a pair of 3-D glasses. I definitely see the person as if in real life, just in front of me. These occurrences have increased through the years in conjunction with the counseling and healing work I have been doing, so my ability to see and communicate more clearly has also developed. I also have to say that, even if you cannot see them, when you are focused on or talking about people who have passed away, since they are not dead, they are attracted to the conversation. Since I do see them, as do quite a few other people, I know that this happens.

At this point in conversation with my clients, in order to confirm my perception, I ask questions. In Joan's case, I asked her if both her grandmothers had passed away, and she said that they had. So I asked the woman who appeared just in front of me as a sort of hazy, ethereal, yet discernable form, if she would say something that her granddaughter would recognize. She said, "Ask her if she remembers about the sweet peas."

So I asked Joan, "Regarding your grandmother, do you remember anything about sweet peas?"

"Oh yes, she grew them every year on vines made of string, and I loved the fragrance."

As Joan said this, I could smell the fragrance of sweet peas around me. At this point, she wanted to talk with her grandmother.

When I realized Joan was open to the fact that her grandmother was present, I let her know her grandmother was there in front of me. Joan wanted to know if her grandmother was the presence she had sensed around herself at times when she experienced great anxiety. At this point, her grandmother said, "Yes, I have been around her at these times, especially when she was anxious over the way her father was treating her and her children." I relayed this message to her, and she responded by breaking into tears, saying she was so grateful to hear this. Joan then told me that her father lives in the same small town, and he is challenged by an addiction to alcohol.

When her grandmother showed up during our session, I immediately got the thought that there was a much more serious issue occurring with Joan than what she had so far disclosed to me. I think that the communication with her grandmother temporarily opened her, and Joan was better able to discuss the issue about her father; her grandmother's question about the sweet peas served to open her up. This gave her the opportunity to ask the question about the sense that her grandmother was around in spirit at times of crises related to her father's abusive behavior; because of this openness, we were able to work together more effectively regarding Joan's relationship with her father.

Our session was about to end at this point, so I asked Joan if there was anything else she wanted to say to her grandmother. She said how grateful she was that her grandmother had shown up and communicated with her this way. I saw that her grandmother heard this, and she indicated to me that she would continue to be around her granddaughter and lovingly support her; I relayed this information to Joan. Then her grandmother slowly faded away from my vision.

Even though people have passed away and are in spirit, what I see when they appear to me is a kind of energy field that forms, and within this field is the image as they looked in their physical bodies in a way that my clients remember, such as in this story, where Joan's grandmother appeared as the elderly woman Joan would recognize.

THE INTENSIVE CARE MANAGER AND HER PARENTS

Sherry was an intensive care unit manager. As we were working together one day, she asked me if I knew anything about seeing people who had passed away. When I told her I did know some things, she said she had experienced seeing the spirit of one of her ICU patients die and leave his body. So now she wanted to know more, and as we talked and I disclosed more of this aspect of my work to her, she asked if I could perhaps talk to her parents.

Just then a woman appeared to me, and she seemed to be Sherry's mother. It is as if those in spirit arrive on the energies of the person's desire who is thinking of them. I said, "Someone is here," as I wanted to confirm who it was and not just assume it was Sherry's mother. I told Sherry that the woman was wearing a dress and had short, curly hair with a hairnet over it. I asked Sherry if this made sense to her. She said, "Yes, that would be my mother. Sometimes her hair was very curly and unmanageable." Those in spirit almost always show themselves in some way or wear something that their loved ones will recognize; they also say certain things, as had the mother who wanted blonde hair.

At this point, I asked Sherry if there was something she would like to ask. She wanted to know how her mother thought Sherry was doing, if her mother ever saw Sherry's dad, and whether the two of them were getting along. Just then a man appeared who seemed to be her father. He showed me that he was doing vegetable gardening, which I told Sherry, and she said that her father liked to garden. She then asked me to ask her parents how they saw her own life moving along. She had had some difficulties with a man she had been involved with for a few years, and she wanted confirmation from her parents that she was doing the right thing by moving away from this man. They actually both encouraged her to find her own place.

Sherry's parents communicated to me that they thought it would be best for Sherry to move out. Those in spirit think the thought rather than say the words, and I receive the thought. They also use body language at the same time, such as waving a hand to indicate what they are trying to communicate. In this case, Sherry's mother and father communicated with gestures and thoughts that their daughter could find someone better for herself. Her mother also gestured a hug toward her daughter, and I communicated this to her.

Sherry burst out in tears after this communication. People who have passed into spirit most often have a wider overview of situations than we do when we are in the midst of living physical life. They want to help because of the connections they have with their loved ones still here. However, just because someone has passed away does not mean they have all-knowing wisdom, but they do very often have a greater overview of life than many people who are living on earth!

This kind of communication, which I enjoy helping to facilitate between loved ones, gives my clients great comfort, as they learn they are not all alone. It also broadens their understanding that much more is going on than what we can see in the physical world. They feel more connected once they have heard from a departed mother, father, or other person close to them. Most people believe in angels, guides, or spiritual masters. I think this belief helps the communication between loved ones here and in spirit, because if there were no belief, I do not think those who are on the other side would even try. Also, people take a wider perspective of their loved ones once they know they are alive in spirit; people see them beyond the personality they remember, and this also makes a difference in people's view of their own lives.

THE MAN WHO WANTED TO KNOW ABOUT HIS GENETICS

This case involved Carl, who heard from a friend of his about my ability to communicate with those who are in spirit. The case was unique and somewhat more interesting to me than others because Carl transcribed his session and sent it to me. He had asked me if I would communicate things to him about his relatives' lives that might have affected his own life through genetic inheritance. For example, his paternal grandmother came to me during our conversation. I learned who she was after asking a few questions to make sure, and he confirmed the answers from her. Here are the relevant parts of Carl's transcribed session.

SHANNON MCRAE: Hello, are you ready to start?

CARL: Yes.

SM: How may I help you?

C: I would like to understand more about my family heritage and some of the incidents in my ancestors' lives that may influence somewhat who and how I am today, genetically, emotionally. I'd like to ask my father's mother, as I remember her the most.

SM: Okay. (Brief pause.) The first image I get is of a woman with a sort of basket or laundry basket; the kind people used to put apples in. They were kind of cumbersome to carry, but almost every woman had one or two or three of them around. Some of the slats are broken.

C: Yes, I remember my grandmother having baskets like these.

SM: Well, she is showing me that she is very frustrated. Did she live on a farm?

C: Yes, both in Lithuania, until she was sixteen, and in the US, in the Midwest, until she married.

SM: And, as a little girl, was she made to work on the farm?

C: I don't know, but she probably did have to. I know her brothers and sisters, who were younger than her, worked hard on the farm.

SM: Okay. She is showing me that she was frustrated because she was made to work, even as a little girl, and it was cold. She has a bonnet because of the cold, but she has no mittens or gloves on her hands. She is saying she is too small and she is made to carry this big basket, and it is too much trouble for her. She just wants to get back to the house where it is warm. She is walking along saying "I will never . . . " as if she resolved to never do this if she could figure out how. And it looks like this resolution has stuck in the DNA passage from her to your father and you a little. It's not you the personality talking, but it is a little in your genetics, your DNA talking, to the point where you will say "I won't ever," or "never will I."

C: I know that I do this a bit. I did it when I was made to work hard. I decided not to ever work hard, but I did anyway.

SM: She had a hard life. She is telling me, "I wanted to read books, but I could never get enough of them to keep myself occupied." She would have to hide to read books, because she was expected to participate on the farm. It was more important to her to go off in a corner somewhere and read for knowledge. And she did get a lot of knowledge. . . . Is there anything else you want me to ask her?

C: I love to read, too. I would often go off and read, away from friends or family. I want to know things like this, and what I could know of her and other family members that she knows of, and their influences, and what might have been passed along to me, to my siblings, to my father.

SM: Okay. (Pause.) She is showing me that she had an uncle—either an uncle or a male cousin—who told her that she would never get anywhere in life. He did that in such a way as to ridicule her for trying to read books. He had that attitude because women in those days, where she was, were not allowed to do what she was trying to do—to self-educate. She is telling me that her mother was very lenient in many respects, and that her mother protected her from her father. Her mother was the go-between, and the father finally did listen to her mother and let her read books.

C: My memory was that she didn't do well with the English language.

SM: She says she could not read English, but she was excellent at her native language, and she did not want to switch over because she feared she would be not so good at the English language. She says there were too many variables in the English and it was too loose for her; she liked the strictness and the way her native language fell together. Also, when other family members started becoming accomplished in American English, she wasn't a bit happy about that. She was very stubborn. I think she passed on a little bit of that stubbornness to you.

C: I can see that!

SM: Are there any more questions?

C: My main question is about the family and things that stand out that may be part of my heritage, any other things that might be helpful for me to know.

SM: She is showing me a great big red barn, and it is very close. It seems to me as if she painted it. It takes up almost the whole canvas. It is like an oil painting. She is showing it to me, and it takes up so much of the picture that it is difficult to see any grass or hills behind it, or even the sky. The top of the barn starts at the top of the canvas, and the bottom goes to the bottom of the canvas and it also covers the canvas from side to side. And she is showing this to me saying, "This is what I did, and it is what Carl is capable of doing, but he needs to push back the main object of his painting and put peripheral things around it." She is showing me her frustration that she can't read English, and secondly that the barn needs to be pushed back in the picture and details put around it so that it looks like the real thing. She says that sometimes you forget the details, not only in your life, but in your artwork, too. She also says the whole family is very creative.

C: Yes, that is all true. And I do look at the big picture but forget how important the details are sometimes. Little things like smiling at someone when you talk, and so on.

SM: She is saying that she had many a difficult time. She lived with family members from time to time. She had her own bedroom, but it was very noisy outside it. She liked her room and is describing the furniture in it and how she enjoyed it, the crystal knobs on the drawers and the carved headboard on the bed. She would go to her room for refuge a lot because she felt like she wasn't wanted or needed, so she would go there to write and read. On warm days, she says, she could go outdoors and paint. She also says she did not have a satisfying relationship with her husband. She says that for a while she tried to make it look like it was satisfying, but it didn't work. She says, "I know it didn't work." So your father grew up in that influence to an extent.

C: Yes. True.

SM: She didn't like small talk at all, anyway.

C: No, she did not, for sure, and neither do I.

SM: She is saying, "I learned to do a lot of things when I was younger." She says she now travels between dimensions to check up on other family members. . . . I just asked her if she believes in the eternality of life, and she told me to "stop the big words!" She says, "It's important that people realize that you keep on living, and there is no change when you keep on living, except that you don't have your body to move around in anymore." She says, "Sometimes the body is cumbersome, but sometimes it's more fun to have a body than to not have a body." She is telling me to tell you to take good care of your body.

She is showing me how rays come out from the sun, like in kids' pictures, and that you can leap from one line to another, but you can't do that when you have a body (she laughs). She is not limited at all in her thinking, yet in some respects she is rigid. She is showing me a picture of a child's drawing of the sun, and when she was a little girl she used to pretend to go out on different rays of the sun and then jump from one to another. And she never stopped pretending to do that. That is where she would go when she got upset or hurt. She would jump to one of those lines coming out, from one to another. She says that is very, very similar to what happens when you make your crossing. She said you read about it and you hear about it, but until you do it you don't understand the mechanics behind it. She says you will hear people say that they reformed their bodies after dying and built houses and other things the way they wanted. You can do that here, too, in physical life. You can create your reality here.

C: I believe all that, and look forward to thinking about it more after our session.

SM: I now see a man who appears to be your father. He is apologizing to you for not being an attentive father. He says, "I had my reasons at the time for thinking I was, but I now know I was not." He says, "Do you remember the red scooter?"

C: Yes, I do remember that scooter. In fact, my grandfather used to call me "Scooter."

SM: He says, "I am sorry I took it away from you when I was punishing you. I always felt sorry about that."

C: Hmmm. I can see that. No worries.

SM: He is also showing me a picture of a top, a spinning top, you know?

C: Yes. I remember I played with one when I was a child, one that had many colors on the surface and made a whistling sound.

SM: I haven't seen one of those in years. He is showing me how you used to spin your top for hours, and he says, "You seemed to be so happy when you were playing with your top." He loved watching you do that. He says he would peek in and watch you do that.

He says you loved it, and you loved to make the high-pitched sound with it.

C: It's true. I remember doing that. It was fun and comforting. I loved the spinning colors.

SM: He is now saying, "I wish I could have helped you more with roller skating." He is showing me that you had some falls, and he wishes he could have been there to help you, because you didn't really keep it up very long to get your confidence going, and he felt a regret over that. He says, "I spent as much time with you as I could."

C: I think he did, too. He was very loving.

SM: Yes. Also, he is showing me that he is wearing a very nice rich blue suit. It's not a navy blue, but a lighter shade, and it looks very, very nice on him, and he has a pale blue shirt on, and a tie with stripes on it. He is saying, "I prefer dressing this way now; it makes me feel good."

C: Hmmm. That's funny. I wonder if he is saying that because I teased him when I was a teenager about wearing better clothes!

SM: He is also showing me a hat, like the ones men wore in the '40s. He is saying, "I wore it for a while, but now it's on a hat rack." He also says, "I am very, very proud of you. What you are doing for people is huge." I see tears running down his cheeks because he is so touched by the work you do for others; he is commending you for the type of service you are providing for people.

C: Thank you, that makes me cry.

SM: Who was the person who sat in a rocking chair with a shawl over her knees?

C: My grandmother loved her rocking chair.

SM: She is showing me that she used to rock in front of the fireplace. It kept her warm. She had arthritis in her knees and she could put a shawl on and keep warm. She liked those times.

C: She used to have me on her lap a lot—even later, when I was a teenager—and I felt my weight was too much for her. I was a bit embarrassed, too, at that age.

SM: She says, "Well, I put the shawl over my knees, so it should have been alright" (laughs). She says she just enjoyed being with you.

A few days after our session, Carl wrote me this note:

> Dear Shannon,
>
> First of all, it was fascinating to me that you so easily saw my deceased relatives in spirit and heard statements from them that neither you nor anyone else could have known otherwise, since you do not know anything about my family and very little about me. I remember my grandmother's apple baskets clearly.
>
> Since my main interest was in knowing a few things that might help me understand more about myself, I was at first confused as to why my grandmother was talking about herself as a little girl. But after I thought about it, I realized that her early experiences would very well have an effect on her and therefore be passed on, to an extent, genetically. Specifically, I think I have some similarities in that I did feel put-upon to work when I was young, and I determined to find a life where I didn't have to work so hard; also, I do like to retreat to a quiet room to read or be quiet when I feel hurt or when life is too noisy.
>
> The part about not being allowed to read also seems to have a role for me in that I sometimes feel it isn't easy for me to

allow myself to take the time. So her frustration is very helpful information, because it helps me resolve my issue. I think there isn't enough time to read all the things I want to read! I have to get over the time crunch element and remember there are just always choices about how you use your time and to use it doing what you enjoy. I have a thirst for knowledge. I suppose that is true for all of us, but I wonder how much comes from my grandmother's and other ancestors' frustrations of not getting all the knowledge they wanted because of limitations. At any rate, it helped me very much to know this, even if only to assess and be more aware of my own feelings.

I think it is true that I have inherited some stubbornness and rigidity. I know I don't like to be cold or to be told to do things, so I often project, and if I think someone is thinking they want me to do something, even if they aren't, I resist! And I do know I tend to say, "I will never do this. . . ."

Another helpful revelation was the part about the big red barn. At first I thought this had nothing to do with me, but upon reflection, I see that it is very true that I see the big picture and can paint it very well. But along the way to getting there, I prefer to pass over important details, including in social interactions. That very unusual metaphor she used at first confused me, but now I see it as a remarkably perceptive and clever way of saying, "Be respectful of the moment-to-moment process of life as you move toward your goals." That was very helpful.

It is also interesting you mentioned that my grandmother said she had an unsatisfying relationship with her husband, my grandfather. I had heard some things about that from my mother. But now that I think about it, I realize that in the back of my mind I did have a part of me that wondered if my relationship with my mate could be satisfying. It is, but a part of me held back, too. It is almost as if a part of me was protecting myself from being fully there because I thought it might not be fully satisfying, and then I would be hurt. I think this was very helpful.

Some of the phrases sound just like things my grandmother would say. She would verbalize things like that, not in a mean way, but with gentleness and a subtle smile, yet she was very firm. I remember my aunts, her sisters, expressing similar firmness in their expressions, unapologetically. My grandmother definitely did not participate in small talk.

And the mourning she described, well, I can tend to go into that about things, but I suppose we all can, and I surmise that most of us have mourning and depression in our family heritage to one extent or another. Still, it was helpful to hear these things, because it made me think about those aspects of myself and about what I want to do to change them, to be happier and to appreciate the life I have.

I have to think more about her description of death and what she said about taking care of and keeping your body healthy. I need to contemplate more about her comments regarding jumping between the sun's rays, but I can see that it is a useful metaphor for being perceptive in many dimensions of time or space.

I loved my grandmother's description of the sun's rays and using that image as a girl. It makes me think of what Einstein said: "Imagination is more important than knowledge." I still laugh when I think about your question to my grandmother about "eternality" and my grandmother's comment to "stop the big words." I can just hear her saying that.

Then the part with my father was very touching to me. I was thirty-one when he died, and I hadn't gotten to know him as an adult because I had been away from home since college. I loved hearing those simple things he said about taking my scooter away and watching me when I was a child, and how he regretted not spending more time with me. I felt very loved and touched. Also, it was quite humorous that he picked out that bit about wearing the nice suit. After the session, I remembered I used to tease him often, for fun, about his clothing choices. I was Joe College. I always used to tell him to wear nicer jackets and shirts! So it was as if he was letting me know that it was him speaking, because I used to joke with him so much about wearing nicer clothes.

Then, when you referred to my grandmother with the shawl and rocking chair—I just realized in rereading that part how Dad used to smile when he saw my grandmother holding me on her lap. She didn't speak much, but I remember being on her lap as the most valuable communication that took place between us, the feeling of the love and care.

I know this could seem very mundane and surface, but the session was very revealing to me and very helpful. I think you are quite talented, and you are so very light about it, not judgmental, but fun to talk with, and accurate and perceptive, very clear. It impressed me that it didn't take you but a few seconds to "tune in" to my relatives.

I also thank you for answering some very important questions I had about my health in such an immediate way. I am convinced you see very clearly. I asked you if there was anything that could be hidden from you, and you said, "No, not really. I've been that way since I was a child, but I am very careful with it. I don't violate people's privacy or go out of my way to know things about people, but often something will just come to me, and I will know something about people around me in public settings." I can now see how nothing can be hidden from you, even if you don't invade privacy, but that if I ask you about something, I had better be ready for the truth; your ability to know is quite profound. I am amazed at how you are not judgmental about anything.

With love,
Carl

I hope readers enjoy this note from Carl. And regarding his last sentence: actually, I don't think I could do what I do if I were judgmental!

THERE IS NO SEPARATION

We can call on loved ones, think about and invite those who have passed away to be with us, just as we can with those friends and loved ones who are still here. We often tap into the same source as those we admire, as we are all connected in our minds. We can access the same mind as those who are accomplished in the sciences, the arts, and any other field. We can call on people who have certain capabilities and talents to help us do what we want to do, and they will. There is more than meets the eye. I could write about so many other cases, but I think that will have to wait for another book.

Notes

Epigraph: Jalal al-Din Rumi in *The Essential Rumi,* New Expanded Edition, Translations by Coleman Barks with John Moyne, HarperSanFrancisco, 1995, 15.

FOREWORD

Epigraph: Laura Day, *How to Rule the World from Your Couch* (San Jose, CA: Simon & Schuster, 2010), 16.

INTRODUCTION

Epigraph: St. Francis of Assisi, in *Love Poems from God,* trans. Daniel Ladinsky (New York, NY: Penguin Compass, 2002).

PROLOGUE

Epigraph: Lynn Robinson, *Divine Intuition: Your Inner Guide to Purpose, Peace, and Prosperity* (San Francisco, CA: Jossey-Bass, 2013).

CHAPTER 1

Epigraph: Robert Dozor, "Scientific foundations of integrative medicine," in *The Heart of Healing: Inspired Ideas, Wisdom, and Comfort from Today's Leading Voices,* ed. Dawson Church (Santa Rosa, CA: Elite Books), 312.

1. Dana Zohar, *Quantum Self* (New York, NY: William Morrow and Company, 1990).
2. Joyce Whiteley Hawkes, *Cell-Level Healing: The Bridge from Soul to Cell* (Hillsboro, OR: Atria/Beyond Words Publishing, 2006).
3. Ibid.

4. Ibid.
5. Amit Goswami, *How Quantum Activism Can Save Civilization: A Few People Can Change Evolution* (Charlottesville, VA: Hampton Roads Publishing Company, Inc., 2011).
6. Ibid.
7. Todd Ovokaitys, in his foreword to *The Twelve Layers of DNA: An Esoteric Study of the Mastery Within* (Kryon Book Twelve; Platinum Publishing House, 2012), describes a DNA study by Russian physicist Vladimir Poponin in which Poponin measured the polarization and orientation of light waves known as photons in a study chamber. The light waves moved randomly in the experimental chamber. However, when he placed DNA in the chamber, it organized the light waves into a coherent pattern. This suggests that DNA possesses a powerful field that influences the organization of space around it. Poponin then performed a control test by removing the DNA from the lab chamber and measuring the photons again. The photons remained in an organized pattern. This suggests that DNA left a residual effect in the space it had previously occupied. It also suggests that human DNA has a powerful effect on the structure or organizational patterns in space around it. For further information see www.abraham-hicks.com for a book and audio CD titled *The Vortex,* which include four wonderful meditations that assist in focusing on healing and physical wellbeing.
8. Hawkes, *Cell-Level Healing.*
9. Dawson Church, *The Genie in Your Genes: Epigenetic Medicine and the New Biology of Intention* (Santa Rosa, CA: Elite Books, 2007), 72–3.
10. Ibid.

CHAPTER 2

Epigraph: Goswami, *Quantum Activism* (see chap. 1, n. 2).

CHAPTER 3

Epigraph: Shakespeare, *Hamlet*, in *The Oxford Shakespeare*, ed. W. J. Craig (London: Oxford University Press, 1914), 2.2.250. References are to act, scene, and line.

CHAPTER 4

Epigraph: Andrew Weil, *Spontaneous Healing: How to Discover and Embrace Your Body's Natural Ability to Maintain and Heal Itself* (New York, NY: Alfred A. Knopf, 1995).

CHAPTER 5

Epigraph: David Hawkins, *The Eye of the I: From Which Nothing Is Hidden* (Sedona, AZ: Veritas Publishing, 1995).

CHAPTER 6

Epigraph: Shakespeare, Sonnet 23, in *The Sonnets: Poems of Love*, ed. William Burto (New York, NY: St. Martin's Press, 1980).

1. Bruce A. Lipton, *Biology of Belief: Unleashing the Power of Consciousness, Matter, and Miracles* (Santa Rosa, CA: Mountain of Love/Elite Books, 2005), 137.

CHAPTER 7

Epigraph: Steve Jobs, quoted in Walter Isaacson, "American icon," *Time Magazine*, October 17, 2011.

1. Hawkes, *Cell-Level Healing* (see chap. 1, n. 2).

CHAPTER 8

Epigraph: Valerie Hunt, *Infinite Mind: Science of the Human Vibrations of Consciousness* (Malibu, CA: Malibu Publishing, 1995).

CHAPTER 9

Epigraph: Leigh Fortson, *Embrace, Release, Heal: An Empowering Guide to Talking about, Thinking about, and Treating Cancer* (Boulder, CO: Sounds True, Inc., 2011).

CHAPTER 10

Epigraph: Robert Holden, *Be Happy!: Release the Power of Happiness in You* (New York, NY: Hay House, Inc., 2009).

CHAPTER 11

Epigraph: Eric Maisel, *Rethinking Depression: How to Shed Mental Health Labels and Create Personal Meaning* (Novato, CA: New World Library, 2012).

peutic touch as energy exchange: Testing the theory,"
ence 6, no. 2 (Jan. 1984): 42–49.
Pain Relief: Dr. Tick's Breakthrough Strategies to Manage
vato, CA: New World Library, 2013).

Epigraph: Ralph Waldo Emerson, *Natural Abundance: Ralph Waldo Emerson's Guide to Prosperity*, ed. Ruth L. Miller (Hillsboro, OR: Atria Books/Beyond Words Publishing, 2011).

1. Melissa Healy, "To prevent stroke injury, sing, dance, touch, look, move?", *Los Angeles Times*, Nov. 17, 2011.
2. Jane Austen, *The Illustrated Letters of Jane Austen*, ed. Penelope Hughes-Hallett (New York, NY: Clarkson Potter Publishers, 1990).
3. Goswami, *Quantum Activism* (see chap. 1, n. 2).

CHAPTER 13

Epigraph: Rabia, in *Love Poems from God*, trans. Daniel Ladinsky (New York, NY: Penguin Compass, 2002).

1. Bob Toben and Fred Alan Wolfe, *Space-Time and Beyond* (New York, NY: Bantam Books, 1982).
2. David Bohm, interview with Renée Weber, "Of matter and meaning: The super-implicate order," *ReVision*, Spring, 1983.
3. *Brain/Mind Bulletin*, 8, no. 12/13.
4. Sir Arthur Eddington, *The Nature of the Physical World* (Cambridge, UK: Cambridge University Press, 1928), 276–77.
5. "Science and technology" (interview with Candace Pert), *Woman of Power*, No. 11 (1988).

CHAPTER 14

Epigraph: Ralph Waldo Emerson, *Self-Reliance and Other Essays*, ed. Stanley Applebaum (Mineola, NY: Dover Publications, 1993).

1. Max Planck, in *Spontaneous Healing of Belief: Shattering the Paradigm of False Limits*, Gregg Braden (New York, NY: Hay House, 2008), 229.

CHAPTER 15

Epigraph: Bill Tomes, quoted in Dan Millman and Doug Childers, *Bridge between Worlds: Extraordinary Experiences That Changed Lives*, (Novato, CA: New World Library, 2009).

1. Bernard Haisch, *The Purpose-Guided Universe: Believing in Einstein, Darwin, and God* (Pomptom Plains, NJ: The Career Press, 2010).

CHAPTER 16

Epigraph: Belinda Gore, *The Ecstatic Experience: Healing Postures for Spirit Journeys* (Rochester, VT: Bear & Company, 2009).

1. For more information on how emotions affect molecules, see Candace Pert, *Molecules of Emotion: The Science behind Mind-Body Medicine* (New York, NY: Touchstone, 1999).

CHAPTER 17

Epigraph: Betty Smith, *Joy in the Morning* (New York, NY: Harper & Row, 1963).

CHAPTER 18

Epigraph: Eckhart Tolle, *Guardians of Being: Spiritual Teachings from Our Dogs and Cats* (Novato, CA: New World Library, 2009).

1. Kelly A. Turner's website for cases of unexpected remission: http://www.unexpectedremission.org.
2. B. O'Regan, *Spontaneous Remission: An Annotated Bibliography* (Institute of Noetic Sciences, 1995).
3. Kelly A. Turner, "When cancer disappears: The curious phenomenon of 'unexpected remission,'" *Noetic Now*, 17 (Dec. 2011), http://www.noetic.org/noetic/issue-seventeen-december/unexpected-remission/.
4. Ibid.
5. Ibid.
6. Ibid.
7. Ibid.
8. Ibid.
9. Ibid.
10. Gregg Braden, "Heart intelligence" (video), http://www.greggbraden.com/.

11. Ibid.
12. Ibid
13. Ibid
14. Institute of HeartMath, see http://www.heartmath.org.
15. Braden, "Heart intelligence."
16. Ibid

CHAPTER 19

Epigraph: Alexis Carrel, *The Voyage to Lourdes* (New York, NY: Harper & Brothers, 1950).

1. Larry Dossey, *Space, Time & Medicine* (Boston, MA: Shambhala Publications, Inc., 1982).

CHAPTER 20

Epigraph: Trevor Campbell, quoted in William Whitecloud, *The Magician's Way* (Novato, CA: New World Library, 2009).

1. Bohm, "Of matter and meaning" (see chap. 13, n. 2).

CHAPTER 21

Epigraph: Ram Dass, *Be Love Now: The Path of the Heart* (New York, NY: HarperOne, 2010).

CHAPTER 22

Epigraph: Anita Moorjani, Dying to Be Me: My Journey from Cancer, to Near Death, to True Healing, New York, NY: Hay House, Inc., 2012).

CHAPTER 23

Epigraph: Rabindranath Tagore, "Stray birds (CIX)," in *Collected Poems and Plays of Rabindranath Tagore* (New York, NY: Macmillan, 1974).

1. Rupert Sheldrake, notes from the Electric Universe Conference, Albuquerque, New Mexico (news release), January 2013, available at: www.sheldrake.org.
2. Gregg Braden, *Spontaneous Healing of Belief: Shattering the Paradigm of False Limits* (New York, NY: Hay House, Inc., 2008), 129.

CHAPTER 24

Epigraph: Carl Jung, in *The Collected Works of C. G. Jung*, vol. 10 (London: Routledge & Kegan Paul, 1964), 164.

CHAPTER 25

Epigraph: Rachel Naomi Remen, quoted in Bill Moyers, *Healing and the Mind* (New York, NY: Broadway Books, 2002).

1. Eckhart Tolle, *The Power of Now: A Guide to Spiritual Enlightenment* (Vancouver, BC: Namaste Publishing, Inc., 1997).

CHAPTER 26

Epigraph: Jerry and Esther Hicks, *Getting into the Vortex: Guided Meditations Audio and User Guide* (New York, NY: Hay House, Inc., 2010).

CHAPTER 27

Epigraph: Hafiz, in *Mala of the Heart: 108 Sacred Poems*, ed. Ravi Nathwani and Kate Vogt (Novato, CA: New World Library, 2010).

1. Max Planck, "The mystery of our being," in *Quantum Questions: Mystical Writings of the World's Great Physicists*, ed. Ken Wilber (Boston, MA: Shambhala Publications, Inc., 1984).

EPILOGUE

Epigraph: Hebrews, 12:1 ESV.

1. Theresa Caputo, "How Talking to the Dead Can Keep You Healthy," episode from The Dr. Oz Show, originally aired September 29, 2014. Available at: http://www.doctoroz.com.

Index

A

Absolute, vi
abuse, 54–56, 184–85
acceptance, 108–9, 174
adrenal glands, 62
Alexander, Eben, 1
alignment
  to purpose, 81
  with Source, 177
  to well-being, 18–19, 107, 109, 136, 161
allergies, 169
American Holistic Medical Association, xii
American Theosophist, The (periodical), xix–xx
anatomy, 31
aneurysm, 29–30
anger, 80, 139
anxiety, 82
appreciation
  health effects from, 97–99, 135
  as high-frequency vibration, 93
  invigorating DNA, 93–94
art, 182
attention, seeking, 70–71, 167
auras, 4
Austen, Jane, 91

B

Be Happy (Holden), 75
beliefs
  causing disease, 165
  changing, 57–59, 166–67
  formation of, 57–59, 126
  healing and, 132–34
  as limiting, 35, 56, 112
  power of, 54
Be Love Now (Ram Dass), 155
bio-fields, 4
blockages
  to flow of well-being, 20
  forgiveness and, 138–39
  illness as, 132
  thought and emotion as, 91–92
blood tests, 166
body/mind/spirit healing, 132–33
Bohm, David, 97, 152
boundaries and boundary issues
  around thoughts, 182–83
  in family relationship, 185–86
  on perceptions, 193–94
  sensitivity and, 186
  in social interactions, 187–88
Braden, Gregg, 133–36
brain
  chemical releases and, 134–35
  consciousness outside, 136
  injury, 47–48

brain fog, 85
Breakthrough to Creativity (Karagulla), xix–xx, 50
Buddy's Candle (McRae), xv

C

Campbell, Trevor, 149
cancer
  appearance of cells in, 39–40, 90
  breast, 34–35, 137–39, 159–61, 185
  conditions of, 132
  depression and, 86–88
  emotions and, 91
  of mole, 90–91
  prevention of, 174–76
  remission of, 131–34
  skin, xviii, 90–91, 101–3, 106–11
  sugar and, 180
  uterine, 26–27
  visualization in healing, 26–27
Cancer Ward (Solzhenitsyn), xv
Capra, Fritjof, xix
Caputo, Theresa, 189–90
Carrell, Alexis, 141
case studies
  of depression, 86–88
  of self-forgiveness, 137–39
  of stress, 64–67
Cayce, Edgar, 6–7, 13–14, 45
cells
  cancer, 39–41
  dark, 65–66
  dysfunctional, 66
  formation of, 143
  healing at level of, 16–22, 24–27, 31–32, 150–51
  intelligence of, 64, 152–53
  light of, 151–52
  from Source field, 25–26
  visualizing, 35, 64
change, embracing, 49–50, 74
Church, Dawson, 26–27, 62
coherence, xiv, 133–39
colitis, 137–38
Collected Works of C. G. Jung, The (Jung), 169
communication, with dead, 10–11, 192–95
compassion, 27–28, 56
complaint, 181
consciousness
  cells influenced by, 64
  controlling matter, 112
  creating quantum possibilities, 21
  measurement and, 184
  as nonlocal, xiv
  as one with the body, 98–99
  outside the brain, 136
  primacy of, 18
cortisol, 46, 62
criticism, 54–57, 93–94
crying sessions, 177–78
cyst, 115–16

D

dark cells, 65–66
Day, Laura, xi
death and dying, 189–91
deceased people
  appearance of, 198–200
  communication with, 10–11, 192–97, 209
  in near-death experience, 190–91
  wider viewpoint of, 201–2
dementia, 186
depression
  case study of, 86–88
  negative thinking and, 83–84
  treatment of, 82, 84–85
depth psychology, xiv
DHEA, 135
disappearing face, 107, 110–11

disease/dis-ease
causes of, 33–35, 91–92, 119
DNA and, 21–22
emotional freedom from, 111
as friend, 104–5
memories and, 67–71
seeking attention with, 70–71, 167
stress and, 38, 53, 160
distant healing, 62, 82, 115, 126, 142, 144–45
Divine Intuition (Robinson), xvii
DNA. *See also* genes
changing, 93–94
field of well-being and, 20–22
light energy and, 20, 24–25
thoughts affecting, 18–19, 62, 66
Dossey, Larry, xix, 46, 104, 141
Dozor, Robert, 15
dream, living your, 185–86
Dreamhealer (McLeod), 103–4
Dying to Be Me (Moorjani), 159

E

eardrum, 40–41
ecstasy, 119
Ecstatic Experience, The (Gore), 119
Eddington, Arthur, 98
EFT. *See* Emotional Freedom Technique
Einstein, Albert, xi, 21
electric currents, 163–64
electromagnetic energies, 179
Embrace, Release, Heal (Fortson), 73
Emerson, Ralph Waldo, 89, 101
Emotional Freedom Technique (EFT), 103, 111, 128–30, 156–57
emotions
affecting molecules, 119
causing disease, 91–92
chronic stress and, 63–67
EFT and, 103, 129–30
healing emotional conditions and, 155–58
releasing, 103, 129–30, 133, 161, 177–78
resolving painful, 124
in social interactions, 187–88
empathy, pain leading to, 43–44
endorphins, 62, 85
energy
channeling, 62, 179
quanta as packets of, 25, 45
energy fields
imbalances in, 51
subtle, 163–64
trauma stored in, 169
energy medicine
basis of, 15–28
effectives of, 52, 81–82
specificity of, 180
term, xix, 50
epigenetic factors, 18, 22, 26
extrasensory perception, 1, 18, 38, 126, 190, 192, 194–95. *See also* higher sensory perception
Eye of the I, The (Hawkins), 49

F

face disappearing in healing, 107, 110–11
failure to thrive, 81
feelings, in healing process, 90, 134–35, 155–58
field
emotional, 69–70, 72
energy, 129, 142, 163
of healing, 17–19, 22–23, 28
of intentional consciousness, 22, 25, 127
quantum, 17, 22, 26, 28, 47, 82, 184
unified or source, 21, 25, 31–33
of well-being, 20–22, 25–28

Field, The (McTaggart), 127–28
5-HTP supplements, 85, 87
focus
  of cancer survivors, 133
  in mending cells, 31–32
forgiveness
  healing power of, 75–80, 138–39
  memories and, 77–79
  process of, 24–25
  of self, 59, 67–68, 129, 156–57, 175–76
Fortson, Leigh, 73
future, foreseeing, xiv

G

GABA (gamma aminobutyric acid), 85, 87
gastroesophageal reflux disease (GERD), 65
genes. *See also* DNA
  potential in, 33–34
  genetic inheritance, 202–13
Genie in Your Genes, The (Church), 26–27, 62
Getting into the Vortex (Hicks and Hicks), 177
goat milk, 127
Gore, Belinda, 119
Goswami, Amit, 18, 29, 94
grandmothers
  of Carl, 202–13
  of Joan, 198–200
  of McRae, 5, 10–11, 192
Guardians of Being (Tolle), 131
gut feelings, 85

H

Hafiz, 181
Haisch, Bernard, 117
Hamlet (Shakespeare), 37
hands, in healing, xii–xiii, 49–50, 89, 146, 179
harmonics, 33–34
Hawkes, Joyce Whiteley, 16–17, 22, 64
Hawkins, David, 49
headaches, 47–48
healers
  as channel of Source energy, 145, 179
  producing energy, 83
healing. *See also* names of diseases
  acceptance of, 108–9
  beliefs and, 132–34
  body/mind/spirit, 132–33
  cellular, 16–22, 24–27, 31–32, 150–51
  crisis, 108–9
  distant, 62, 82, 115, 121, 142, 144–45
  emotions/feelings in, 90, 134–35, 155–58
  field of, 17–19, 22–23, 28
  forgiveness and, 75–80, 138–39
  group, 94
  hands in, xii–xiii, 49–50, 89, 146, 179
  intention in, xv, 17, 23, 106–7
  light and, 107
  mechanics of, 112
  patients participating in, xv, 23–25, 49–50
  place/space, 22–25, 107, 167–68
  potential for, 50–52
  ripple effect of, 158
  self-induced, xv
  spiritual, 103
  at subatomic level, 16–17
  surrender and, 79–80
  unexpected, 137
  visualization and, 22, 26–27, 86–87
  willingness to change and, 49–50
  Worrall and, xii–xiii

Healing and the Mind (Remen), 173
healing process, of McRae, 30–33
health care professionals, 50
heart, coherence and, 134–35
Heart of Healing, The (Dozor), 15
Hebrews 12:1, 189
hepatitis C, 149–53
herbs, 133
Hicks, Esther and Jerry, 177
higher sensory perception, xx–xxi, 1–2. *See also* extrasensory perception
Hill, Napoleon, 165
Holden, Robert, 75
holding space, 107
hospice, 40, 113, 195–98
How to Rule the World from Your Couch (Day), xi
Hunt, Valerie, 69
hyper-intelligence, 12

I

imbalances, in energy field, 51
immune system, 180
Infinite Mind (Hunt), 69
injuries
  examples of, 51–52
  seeking attention with, 70–71
  self-inflicted, 76–78
inner guides, xiii
inner knowing, 125–26
Institute of HeartMath, 135
Institute of Noetic Sciences (IONS), 125, 132
intention
  to feel positive emotions, 133
  in healing, xv, 17, 23, 106–7
  to help, 89–90
  mutual, 23, 28, 71
  power of, 127–28
  in therapeutic touch, 144–45
Intention Experiment, The (McTaggart), 127
interconnectedness
  of body/mind/spirit, 132–33
  at level of quanta, 37, 184
intuition
  in cancer survivors, 133
  definition of, xvii
  as quantum leap, 29
  value of, 53
intuitive insight
  identifying health issues, 53
  illness and, 7
  scanning body with, 120–21
  into thought patterns, 55
isolation, 6–9, 12

J

Jobs, Steve, 61
journaling, 86, 170
joy, 75
Joy in the Morning (Smith), 125
judging
  refraining from, 94–95
  self, 54, 68, 129
  tension caused by, 165
Jung, Carl G., xiv, 169

K

Karagulla, Shafica, xix–xx, 50
kefir, 127
Krieger, Dolores, xix, 103, 144
Kübler-Ross, Elisabeth, 113–14
Kuhlmann, Katherine, 45
Kunz, Dora van Gelder, xix–xx, 103, 144

L

law of attraction, 34, 144

letting go
  to become true self, 173
  effects in body of, 156–57
  in healing process, 73–74, 105–6
  to reach ecstasy, 119
  in self-forgiveness, 67–68
  in transition to death, 196
light energy
  in body, 16, 24–25
  DNA organizing, 20
  healing and, 107
  structuring matter, 98, 152
Lipton, Bruce, 54
listening, nonjudgmental, 114–17
liver, 149–53
Long Island Medium, 189–90
loss, xi
Louis, Roberta, xix
love, 53, 97, 113
Love Poems from God (Rabia), 97
lungs, 145–47

M

Magician's Way, The (Campbell), 149
Maisel, Eric, 81
Mala of the Heart (Hafiz), 181
Master, 12
matter
  mind as matrix of, 112
  primacy of, 18
  quanta as, 16
  as slowed-down light, 152
McLeod, Adam, 103–4
McRae, David, xviii
McRae, Shannon
  childhood of, 1–11
  coloring books and, 4
  deceased appearing to, 10–11, 198–200
  extrasensory perception of, 1–2
  grandmothers of, 5, 10–11, 192
  healing process of, 30–33, 105–7
  hospice work of, 40, 117, 195–98
  illness of, 6–8
  intelligence of, 12
  intuition of, xvii
  isolation of, 6–9, 12
  mother and, 2–9
  near-death experience of, xi–xii, 8–10, 191–92
  out-of-body experiences of, 190–91
  predictions of, 3–4
  as preschooler, 3–4
  silvery beings seen by, xii, 1, 8–10
  unseen helpers and, xiii–xiv
  Worrall healing, xii–xiii
McRae family, 1–12, 192
McTaggart, Lynne, 127
measles, 7
meditation, 15
melatonin, 85, 128
Melvin, Mael, xix
memories
  disease and, 67–71
  forgiveness and, 77–79
  forgotten, 38, 92
milk thistle extract, 153
mind, 98, 112
Mind, as matrix of matter, 112
Miners, Scott E., xvii–xxii
Minister's Manual, The, (McGlone), 113
Mitchell, Edgar, 125
Molecules of Emotion (Pert), 62
monitoring thoughts, 36, 54
Moorjani, Anita, 159
Moss, Richard, 125
music, 182

N

National Institute of Mental Health, 98

Natural Abundance (Emerson), 89
natural remedies, 102–3
Nature, 89, 181–82
naturopathic physicians, 87, 137
NCTT. *See* non-contact therapeutic touch
NDE. *See* near-death experience
near-death experience (NDE)
of McRae, xi–xii, 8–10, 191–92
of Siegel, xi–xii
negative energy, 90–91
negative self-image, 54–59
negative thinking
causing depression, 83–84
coherence and, 137
habitual, 62, 91–92
monitoring, 54
reducing, 34
ways to redirect, 21–22, 165
negative thought, 54–55
neurons, in gut, 85
New Earth, A (Tolle), 123
new life story, 105
non-contact therapeutic touch (NCTT), 81–82, 144–45, 160
nonlocality of consciousness, xiv
nurturing, lack of, 81–83
nutrition, 8, 127

O

OBE. *See* out-of-body experiences
observer effect, 18, 21
obsessive thoughts, 171–72
On Death and Dying (Kübler-Ross), 113
Orbito, Alex, 103
out-of-body experiences (OBE)
of Alexander, 1
of McRae, 190–91
overweight, 129–30
oxytocin, 81–82
Oz, Mehmet, 163, 189–90

P

pain, 43–44, 122–24
pain body, 122–24
paradigm shift, 18
parasite, 115–16
patterns, in symptoms, 178
perception, controlling, 183, 193–94
Pert, Candace, 62, 98, 119
physical body
coherence of, 135–37
consciousness and, 98–99
electromagnetic energy and, 179
emotions and, 119
energy fields and, 163–64
as light waves, 16
as not solid, 37–38, 97
thoughts affecting, 66, 98–99, 165–68
pineal gland, 85
Planck, Max, 112, 181–82
positive outcomes, 62, 142–44
positive thought, 54–55, 86, 141
positive vibrations, 21
potential
in genes, 33–34
for healing, 50–52
in quanta, 45
Pottenger, Jr., Francis M, 8
Pottenger's Cats (Pottenger), 8
Power of Now, The (Tolle), 174
prayer
Dossey books about, 46, 104, 141
effects of, 141–44
Prayer is Good Medicine (Dossey), 141
precognition, xxi, 183
present, being, 114–17, 123
Proof of Heaven (Alexander), 1
protection, 186–88
purpose, 117

Purpose-Guided Universe, The, (Haisch), 117
push buttons, 186

Q

quanta
  as packets, 16, 25
  potentials of, 45
  as unseen energy, 25, 45
Quantum Activism (Goswami), 29
quantum energy, 15–16
quantum field
  distant healing and, 82
  observer effect and, 17–18, 20, 184
  thought creating, 17
quantum physics
  interconnectedness and, 37, 94–95
  particles as waves in, 97
  potentials and, 21, 45
quantum reality, 22, 64
Quantum Self, The (Zohar), 16

R

rabbis, xiii
Rabia, 97
Ram Dass, 155
readiness, 157
relationships, 57, 184–86
releasing. *See* letting go
Remen, Rachel Naomi, 173
remission, 175–76
remote viewing, 38, 46, 120–21
repression, 13
resilience, 173–76
Rethinking Depression (Maisel), 81
rheumatic fever, 6–7, 122–23
Rhine Research Center, 83
ripple effect of healing, 158
Robinson, Lynn, xvii
Rumi, Jalal al-Din, vi

S

St. Francis of Assisi, 1
scanning, 120–21, 143
self-blame, 138
self-disclosure, 121–22
self-esteem, low, 56–57, 70, 129
self-forgiveness, 59, 67–68, 80, 86, 129, 156–57, 175–76
self-induced healing, xv
self-love, 93–94
self-respect, 58–59
self-sabotage, 138–39
self-worth, 53–54, 56
Selye, Hans, 64
separation after death, 213
serotonin, 87
Shakespeare. William, 37, 53
Sheldrake, Rupert, 125
Siegel, Bernie, xi–xvi, xix, 104
silence, 23
silvery figures, xii, 1, 8–10
Simonton, Carl, 26, 35
sinus congestion, 145–46, 177–78, 179–80
Sjogren's syndrome, 120
skin cancer, 82, 101–2, 107–11
Smith, Betty, 125
social interactions, 187–88
solitude, 43
Solzhenitsyn, Alexander, xv
Sonnet 23 (Shakespeare), 53
Source
  energy, 18, 19, 145
  field of well-being, 25–26
space, for healing, 22–25, 107, 167–68
Space, Time & Medicine (Dossey), 141
space-time, 141
spiritual beings, 8–10
spiritual healing, 103
spontaneous healings, 74, 104, 131–34

Spontaneous Remission Project, 132
St. John's Wort, 85, 87
stories, 114
"Stray Birds" CIX (Tagore), 163
stress
  affecting DNA, 21
  causing illness, 33, 38, 53, 160
  chronic emotional, 63–67
  coherence and, 135
  cortisol and, 46
  negative, 62–63
  positive, 62
  thoughts and, 61–63, 103, 126
  unresolved, 61–63
Sugrue, Thomas, 13, 45
super-sensory focus, 120
supplements, 133, 153
surrender
  to healing, 23, 47, 79–80, 106–7
  to present moment, 174

T

Tagore, Rabindranath, 163
tapping technique, 130
Tart, Charles, 125
tears, 80
therapeutic touch, xix, 144–45
Therapeutic Touch movement, 103
There Is a River (Sugrue), 13, 45
Think and Grow Rich (Hill), 165
thought
  affecting body, 98–99, 165–68
  affecting DNA, 18–20, 62, 164
  alignment of, 18–19, 107, 109
  body responding to, 66
  boundary issues around, 182–83
  causing diseases, 91–92
  creating quantum field, 17
  energy of, 164–65
  imprinting on matter, 69
  monitoring, 36
  negative, 54–55
  obsessive, 171–72
  positive, 54–55, 86, 141
  ruling material world, 101
  sensing others, 164–65
  stress and, 61–63, 103, 126
  as vibrations, 19
thyroid, 127–28
Tick, Heather, 85
timeless zone, 110–11
Time Magazine, 61
Tolle, Eckhart, 123, 131, 174
Tolpen, Bob, 97
Tomes, Bill, 113
total health, 104, 111, 174
touch therapies, 81–82
toxins, 177, 180
transition, help with, 196–97
trauma, stored, 169
trust, 121–22
Turner, Kelly A., 131–32

U

unseen helpers, xiii–xiv
unworthiness, 58

V

vibrations
  of appreciation, 93
  positive, 21
  thoughts as, 19
  as wave energy, 33–34
visualization
  of anatomy, 31
  of cells, 35, 64
  in healing, 22, 26–27, 86–87
  by patient, 26–27
  Simonton and, 26, 35
  of subatomic level, 16–17
vitamins, 103, 133

vortex, 23
Voyage to Lourdes (Carrell), 141

W

wave energy, 97
well-being
  alignment of thoughts to, 18–19, 107, 109
  coherence and, 136
  connection to pure, 181–82
  field of, 20–22, 25–28
  as greatest potential, 33
  in healing space, 23
  as positive vibration, 21
  as Source energy, 19
Well Being Journal, xviii–xix, 52
Winfrey, Oprah, 123, 163
Wisdom from World Religions (Templeton), 101
Wolf, Fred Alan, 97
women, in abusive situations, 184–85
Worrall, Olga, xii–xiii
worthiness, 58

X

X-rays, 79

Z

Zohar, Dana, 16